BODY and SOUL
Children, Teenagers and CANCER

MARK RAGG

D1800060

Hill of Content
Melbourne

First published in Australia 1994
by Hill of Content Publishing
86 Bourke Street
Melbourne 3000

© C. Sciacca 1994
© M. Ragg 1994

Cover: Painting *Two Fires in One Flame* by Guy Mirabella
        Design by Guy Mirabella
Printed in Australia by Australian Print Group

National Library of Australia
Cataloguing-in-publication data

Ragg, Mark.
   Body and soul.

   Bibliography
   Includes index.

   ISBN 0 85572 252 5

   1. Tumours in adolescence. 2. Tumours in children.
   3. Cancer. I. Title.
362.1969940083

Contents

Foreword

'He was gentle, kind, caring and considerate. His concern was never for himself, but for others.'

This quote, now engraved on a tombstone in a Brisbane cemetery, encapsulates the driving force and the motivation behind the publication of *Body and Soul.*

We dedicate this book to the memory of the late Sam Sciacca, our son, whose life was tragically cut short at the tender age of nineteen years.

Sam was just a typical young Grade 12 student, who had never had a sick day in his life and who made a point of getting on with people and helping them, rather than involving himself in confrontations and dramas. He was the perfect son—not a brilliant academic or brilliant sportsman but simply a pleasure to have around and someone who was always happy just to be alive and where possible to bring pleasure to other people's lives. Nothing was ever too much trouble for him and everybody with whom he came in contact loved him.

Tragically, out of nowhere, came an enemy that no-one could have foreseen, least of all, Sam himself. After leading a generally healthy life, with the exception of minor colds and flu, he contracted the most terrifying disease of all, cancer. He fought it bravely for seven months until even his own fighting spirit and extraordinary will to live was overcome by the virulence of the bone cancer that struck him, namely Ewing's sarcoma.

Naturally, as a loving family we looked for answers. What was Ewing's sarcoma all about? How was it contracted? What were the treatments? How does a family face such a tragic circumstance? These were questions that we, as a family, found very difficult to obtain answers for. Sure, there were plenty of publications from various cancer organisations which were of help but, after receiving the devastating news that our son had cancer in September 1991, we could find nothing to help us get through the next seven months. It was fear of the unknown, of what it was that we could do, how to handle the situation, how to live whatever time was left with Sam, so that every day would be as enjoyable as it could be, not only for us but for our son.

While there is life, there is hope. No family will ever give up, and naturally we were interested in any treatments, either medical or alternative, that were available. We did all of that and more, but it was always very difficult because of the lack of anything substantive that we could put our hands on that would give us some indication as to what we were facing and how to handle it.

When our son passed away, we racked our brains trying to think of some way to perpetuate his memory and do something which we knew he would want us to do. The idea then came for this book *Body and Soul*, which we hope, and which we know Sam would hope, will be of comfort and assistance to those who may find themselves facing the same circumstances as our family and the very many thousands of others who have lost dear ones, particularly their children, to this terrible disease.

We know that our son would be pleased because it was exactly what he would have done had he been placed in the same position. They say there is a silver lining behind every cloud and perhaps this is the silver lining in the dark cloud of our tragedy in losing our only beloved son.

This book would not have been possible had it not been for the tremendous support and assistance that our family received from people from all walks of life, including Members of the Australian Federal Parliament, State Parliament and local government from all sides of politics and our many hundreds of friends and our dear relatives who encouraged us in this endeavour. We will not mention them by name because they know who they are, but in particular, we wish to thank the author, Dr Mark Ragg, who accepted the commission to write this book on the strict understanding that it would be written in a simple and straightforward manner so that it would be easy reading for anybody that picked it up. Notwithstanding that it deals with many medical issues and contains many medical terms, he has fulfilled his brief extraordinarily well and for that, we thank him.

We hope that this book will be of assistance to many people in the future. While our own story did not have a happy ending, contracting cancer is not a death sentence. With newly emerging technology and drugs improving all the time, there are numerous happy endings. We urge all families and people who find themselves in our position in the future never to give up hope—never stop trying and just in case, always ensure that you live every day at a time and that you treasure and hold dear every second that we are allowed with our loved ones on this earth.

This one is for you, son. We know in our hearts that this is what you would want us to do.

Con, Tina and Zina Sciacca

Introduction

Cancer in children and teenagers is not common. You probably would not have thought it possible before your son or daughter was diagnosed with it. So when confronted with the fact that your child has a serious illness, and you know little or nothing about it, it is hard to know how to cope.

The aim of this book is to help you cope. You will be able to deal better with the pain, the frustration, the fears and the anxiety of cancer if you have more idea what it all means.

Body and Soul exists only because of the efforts of Con and Tina Sciacca, of Brisbane. Their son Sam was diagnosed with Ewing's sarcoma, a rare bone cancer, in September 1991. Sam died on 13 April 1992, aged 19. Con and Tina realised that one problem they faced during that time was the lack of information available to patients. There was a bit of information in medical textbooks on Ewing's sarcoma, but very little that non-medical people could read.

So they established the Sam Sciacca Foundation and

raised money to help people with Ewing's sarcoma. Their main effort has been to commission me to write this book, and they will distribute copies of *Body and Soul* to libraries and hospitals throughout Australia. They hope that because of their efforts, parents of children and teenagers with cancer will know a little more about what lies ahead.

Body and Soul has three parts. The first deals with all the things you might not think to ask your doctor. How will the cancer affect our lives? Our other children? Our relationship? What special needs do teenagers have? What if our child is dying?

These questions are equally as important as the questions about the physical impact of the cancer, but too often they are neglected. Because the child with cancer is not alone. The child with cancer is part of a family. When a child has cancer, everybody in the family is affected. Everybody.

The second part contains interviews with some people who had survived cancer, and some families of those who did not. Because of Con and Tina's special interest, I specifically interviewed people who had had Ewing's sarcoma. But the information contained is relevant to everyone with cancer.

When you read these, I don't want you to think: 'Oh, this is what's going to happen.' All the interviews are different, and all the experiences of those involved are different. Some of the things these families discuss might happen to you, others will not. But the aim is to allow you to see what might lie ahead. The assistance of those who spoke to me is greatly appreciated, and their stories are really the core of this book. For this book to be of any use, it has to be about people, not statistics.

The third part deals with the nuts and bolts of Ewing's sarcoma. Who gets it? Why? What treatment is available? What side effects might my child get? What are his or her chances of survival? All the questions that you want to ask your doctor, but might not.

Although some of the information in this part is specific to Ewing's sarcoma, much of it is relevant to all children and teenagers with cancer. So read it, and ignore the bits that don't apply to you and your child.

Body and Soul is written as if you are reading it the day after your son or daughter was diagnosed with cancer. That may not be true. He or she may be halfway through the course of treatment. Or may have finished the course of treatment. Or may have died. Or you may just suspect he or she has cancer, and you want to find out all you can about it. That's fine, just read on. From wherever you are, this book will provide information on what is ahead, and explain what has already happened.

Although *Body and Soul* was written for parents of people with cancer, I hope everybody can read it—people with cancer, friends and family. Understanding what is going on is half the battle in conquering fears and dealing with difficult issues.

Mark Ragg

Acknowledgements

Many, many people have helped with the compilation of this book. My thanks to:

Doreen Akkerman; Dr John Allman; Dr Geoff Beadle; Diane, Jessie and Don Bond; Mark Bretherton; Phillipa Butters; Rhonda, Alan and Lauren Cameron; Michael Carr-Gregg; Dr Marylon Coates; Dr Penny Cousens; John Dean; Dr Stuart Dunn; Dr J. Dunst; Jan, Lisa and Tricia Griffin; Christina Hardy; Professor Jun-ichi Hata; Sue Hearn; Senator John Herron; Professor Herbert Jurgens; Joyce Kelly; Janet, Frank and Bruce Knight; Professor Bill Marsden; Patrick, Sue and Brian McCabe; Dr Stan McCarthy; Sue Murray; Professor Darcy O'Gorman Hughes; Kathy and Paul Price; Greg Rudd; Rhondda Rytmeister; Dr Helen Somerville; Bruce Warren; Freda and Vanessa Wengert; Anne-Louise, Christine and Ray Van Den Nieuwenhof; and Corinne, Pauline, Chris and Rod Woollard. Doubtless there are others whom I have left out.

In particular, I would like to acknowledge my debt to Christina Brock and George Kannourakis for suggestions and help with the manuscript. Any outstanding errors are all mine.

I would like to thank Gayle Stone for her support throughout the period of research and writing, and thank Con and Tina Sciacca for their drive to get this book published.

I would also like to acknowledge the bravery and honesty of all those I interviewed about how the cancer affected their lives. A lot of tears fell during the telling, and the typing, of those stories.

PART 1

Soul—
what the books say

Parents

Your child has cancer. How do you, as parents, feel? What should you do? How will you cope?

It seems all parents initially react the same. Shock comes first, the terrible shock of 'why my child?' There seems to be no good reason for it, and there is not. There is no childhood cancer where doctors can say 'this is what caused it'. Although doctors are looking for causes, all they are finding is vague associations.

Along with that shock is the fear that your child will die. Although something like 75–80 per cent of all children with cancer will be cured, most people still strongly associate cancer with death. So when you first hear that your child has cancer, it is natural to immediately think he or she is going to die.

In many cases, this shock and grief is similar to the period of mourning after the death of someone you have loved. The only difference is that parents are mourning the possible death of their child, rather than the actual death.[1]

Sometimes this is a good thing. It allows parents to

3

think about life without their child and lets them deal with some of their emotions so they can later concentrate on helping their child through treatment. It also helps parents adjust if the child dies quickly.

But there can be problems if the parents thoroughly mourn for their child and the child survives. The parents have adjusted themselves to life without their child, then they must readjust back. It can be quite difficult and professional help, such as from a psychologist, may be needed.

After that initial shock and period of what is called anticipatory mourning, almost anything can happen. Some parents become very angry, some deny the existence of the cancer, some turn to God, some feel that in some way they are responsible for their child's illness. About half become either depressed or anxious, although these feelings usually ease up some time during the treatment.

Some throw themselves wholeheartedly into searching for cures, reading medical journals, hunting out alternative treatments and devoting their lives to the hope of a cure. Others place all their faith in their doctors and become passive recipients of what the system has to offer.

The only common thread is that if the child enters remission, most parents start to feel increasing hope that all will be well. It can be a period of great uncertainty, as there is no set period after which doctors say 'right, you're cured!' It is simply that each day without cancer slightly lessens the chance of it coming back.

A relapse can be devastating. Many parents find their child's relapse harder to take than the initial diagnosis, because they know by now that it is that bit harder to treat cancer second time around than it was first time.[1] They also know what is ahead of them.

Rearing your child while all this is going on

The traditional advice is: 'treat your child as normally as possible'. That makes sense. You want your child to grow up normally, and you want this experience with cancer to be just a part of growing up, so it makes sense to treat a child with cancer as you would treat any other child.

The trouble is that it can be unbelievably difficult to do. Most parents, even though they want to treat their child normally, are overprotective and overindulgent. They are torn between wanting to see their child as normal, and wanting to provide everything they can in what they worry may be their child's last few months or years. As well, they have to deal with all the things they would never have been prepared for—fear, their child's pain and suffering, talking about cancer and death. Again, many parents need or would benefit from professional help to deal with being parents.

When the child is a teenager

The particular difficulty facing a family in which a teenager has cancer is that the former child is in the process of moving away from the family. A parent or a younger child knows his or her place—the teenager is in a state of turmoil. He or she wants independence, but does not yet have it. Even the independence of being able to travel on his or her own may not yet have been granted.

Parents who had begun to let go may find that they revert to their former protective selves. They start picking up on their child's eating habits, dress, friends, social activities and sleeping patterns—concerns they may have eased up on some time earlier.[2]

The reason for these concerns is quite obvious— parents who are used to being able to control the lives of their children suddenly find that they can control very little. They can't control the cancer, or the treatment, or the hospital. Their own lives are in turmoil because of the threat of death to their child, the demands of time and money placed on them by treatment, and the guilt they feel that somehow they have contributed to their child's illness.

So they respond by trying to control what they can control—how much their son eats, whether their daughter gets enough sleep and so on. Often the main conflicts between parents and children are over minor matters such as these, when real issues such as death and fears and hopes and treatments go silently by.

The problem is that this impedes the growth and development of the teenager, as well as destroying lines of communication between parent and child that need to be open. It also harms the teenager's ability to adapt to his or her disease.[2] As well, it enhances the difficulties facing the teenager who is feeling like he or she has little control over life. If a parent tries to impose order, that will only add to the teenager's sense of helplessness.

Demands

Having a sick child places enormous demands on parents. It is a financial burden in many ways. One parent or both may have to give up work or cut back on hours worked so as to be with the child more often and be available for trips to the hospital and doctors. Your sick leave will be consumed very quickly. Many people who regularly work overtime find they have to give that up to be more available for their child. An American study has found that this burden usually falls on the mother—45 per cent of women said their work was significantly interrupted compared to 20 per cent of men.[3]

Although treatment under Medicare is provided free

of charge, there can be many other expenses that do not count as strictly medical and are not covered by Medicare. These include sheepskin underlays if your child is spending long periods in bed, special foods and vitamin supplements if required, and a million other gadgets and gizmos to help your child. As well, travelling to and from hospitals and surgeries can be expensive.

You will have to grapple with concepts you had not considered before. Doctors will explain the risks and benefits of having a particular test or form of treatment, and expect you to have a say in deciding what to do. You will feel lost because of the names of the drugs, the length of the treatment and the uncertainty of the outcome. You will wonder whether you have done the right thing.

You will have to cope with what is an enormous disruption to your normal family life. Instead of attention being shared equally throughout the family, it is focused on the sick child. Instead of having mealtimes together to talk about the day's events, they can be broken up with hospital visits. Instead of being able to plan ahead for day trips or holidays, you will be able to plan little until treatment is over and your child is regaining his or her health.

You will have to watch your child suffer. You will wonder, perhaps many times, whether the pain and disruption and indignity caused by the treatment is any better or worse than the cancer itself. You will feel guilty that it is your decision to make the child go through treatment, yet you cannot share any of the pain caused by that decision. You will wonder whether it is all worth it. Yet you will almost certainly decide to continue treatment because the hope that your child will live is stronger than anything else.

You will experience different problems at different times. For example, one of the first problems you will face is dealing with the health system, which is complex. There will seem to be too many people telling you what to do, and making suggestions, and pulling your child this way and that. You will feel that you would like to protect your child from all this, but you know you will not be able to do so. Having a family doctor whom you trust can be very helpful.

You will feel exhausted by trying to keep up all your normal activities—work, within home or outside, looking after other children, some sort of social life—while coping with this additional burden of a sick child. This is particularly so while your child is in hospital.

Even after treatment is over, you will find it hard to plan anything with certainty. This will make it hard for you to take a holiday, change jobs, decide to have another child, move house, or change anything significant in your life.

You will find that your life is focused on one day at a time, and you might find it hard to look to the future.

You will also find that you want to suppress your feelings. You will try to hide your true fears and frustrations and hopes from your child, and perhaps from your partner.

Most parents cope with all these demands. However it is hard, and problems can occur. Typically they show up as trouble sleeping, drinking too much, difficulties at work or in the marriage, and feeling isolated.

Although parents react in a variety of ways, research has suggested that some common themes emerge. These are:[4]

- parents are unprepared for the diagnosis. They put the symptoms down to something minor, like a bruise or a cold;
- they initially give all control to the doctors and hospital, although later they want to regain control;
- they are given enough information to deal with in the early days, but later demand more information;
- their methods of dealing with statistical information, such as the chances of survival, vary enormously;

- they are scared about bringing the child home;
- they need to maintain as normal a family life as possible;
- they tend to devalue their local doctor and rely on specialists;
- they are terrified of a recurrence;
- the eventual death of a child after a prolonged illness often brings a sense of relief;
- parents find anniversaries of diagnosis or death stressful;
- they fear other children will develop cancer;
- they find it hard to deal with other children;
- they feel isolated—they think nobody understands what they are going through.

Problems for families of people with cancer

Initial phase
   Managing emotional tensions
   Feeling excluded from the focus of care
   Communicating with staff
Adaptation phase:
   Adjusting to changes in roles and lifestyles
   Meeting the needs of other family members
   Living with uncertainty and with others
Terminal phase:
   Communicating about death
   Providing care and support to the dying
   Dealing with separation and loss

Source: Northouse L. The impact of cancer on the family: an overview. *International Journal of Psychiatry in Medicine* 1984; **14**: 215–42.

Effects on your marriage

It used to be thought that having a child with cancer was enough to break up a marriage. In one way that's true, in another way it is not.

On the one hand, there is evidence that a serious illness puts great strains on a marriage, and that these strains can make a couple think about splitting up.

On the other hand, divorce rates show a couple of things. They show that overall some couples get divorced earlier than they would have—for example, a couple who would probably get divorced after fifteen years may do so after ten years because of the strain of dealing with cancer.[5] But they also show that overall, roughly the same number of couples who have a child with cancer divorce as other couples. If anything, it might be even less.

A simple way of looking at it is this. If your marriage is strong then having cancer in your family will create a few problems, but will not cause a divorce. If your marriage is weak, a child with cancer may hurry its end.

The message is that your marital relationship needs work. Raising a child is hard enough work, so raising a child with cancer and going through the treatment is naturally going to be even harder. All your efforts to help each other and support each other and give each other time will need to be doubled. It would also help if you could occasionally pass the responsibility for your sick child to somebody else and have time together.

Effects on the family

The effect on the family unit is difficult to work out. One study found that the cancer experience often strengthens the family unit, where friends and acquaintances who have more distant ties can avoid or abandon the person with cancer. In a way, it is a period of sorting out who are your real friends and who are not.[6]

Another used psychological testing to examine the impact of childhood cancer on the family. It found that mothers scored as if they were clients of stress management clinics, and had lower than normal self-esteem. Oddly, fathers had higher than normal self-esteem. Marriages were under pressure—they were worse than average but better than divorced couples. Children reported higher than normal levels of conflict within the home.[7]

A third found that families of cancer survivors were not, at higher risk of psychological distress or family problems than average, although these did occur in families with little social support. Social support buffered the effect of chronic strain or depression in fathers and anxiety in mothers.[8]

A consistent finding from many studies has been the impact on other children. See the following chapter Brothers and Sisters for details on that.

Brothers and Sisters

Sibling relationships—relationships between brothers and sisters—can be the longest relationships of a person's life. Parents eventually die, friends come and go, but a brother is always a brother and a sister is always a sister until death do you part.

Sibling relationships can be very intense, especially in early childhood. Siblings can exert a strong influence on the developing personality of each other—they can be teacher, comforter, supporter, enemy, friend and protector. Sibling relationships are full of love, hate, jealousy, rivalry, betrayal, deceit, loyalty, cruelty and support.[1]

So anything that happens to one child affects your other children.

The impact on the sibling

Think of it this way. Every fear, every ache, every pain, every worry and every hope that you experience, your

12

children are feeling, too. That is not just the child with cancer, but that child's brothers and sisters. Dealing with cancer is not easy for anybody, and siblings of children with cancer find it just as hard as parents.

Siblings face a good deal of separation from their family and friends. They may miss a lot of school. In most families, the mother may spend most of her time at the hospital while the father takes over many of the home duties. They may be farmed out to grandparents and neighbours and friends. The routine certainties of their lives are disrupted. Their emotional needs are often neglected, and the long-term planning most parents typically undertake for schooling and socialisation may also be ignored. The common response from parents is that they will worry about the needs of the sibling 'later', when the sick child is either cured or has died.[1]

But what little research has been done has showed that siblings suffer greatly during this period of illness. On psychological scales, they are even more distressed than the sick child or the parents. They feel their parents have stopped speaking to them and they have no control over what is happening.[2]

A common finding is that siblings often do not know what is going on. They know their brother or sister is sick, but they do not know the full extent of the illness. They are not told about treatments and they are rarely given an understanding of whether their sibling is dying or not. In fact, many are surprised when they realise their brother or sister is about to die. As well, if parents trivialise the illness, they can feel terribly confused. They can see their brother or sister looking sick, lying in hospital unable to come home, but their parents tell them not to worry about it.[2]

Their home often doesn't feel like a home any more. If the child with cancer is in hospital for long periods, then months can pass between routine dinners where all the family sits together. They often complain that it is lonely and sad at home.

They may feel their parents are treating them unfairly. They are expected to take on more of the responsibilities of home and act more maturely—whether that be washing up or mowing lawns or putting away toys or learning to iron—yet parents rarely have the time or energy to show their appreciation of this attempt to grow up rapidly. As well, they may be treated differently to the sick child. If they have an argument, as brothers and sisters tend to do, then it is likely they will be blamed for causing trouble. The sick child, consciously or unconsciously, is usually favoured by the parent. He or she may well be manipulating that situation.

Siblings can feel or exhibit any number of responses to these stresses. Their behaviour can suffer—they may start to avoid school, or avoid the hospital, or take up bed-wetting or soil their pants, or start fires. They can suffer any number of physical symptoms such as headaches and abdominal pains. They can feel anxiety and rejection. Their relationships with their parents can suffer. They can feel isolated and left out.[1] At times, they might say they wished their brother or sister would hurry up and die. Then they feel guilty that they were thinking that way.

Younger siblings can have particular problems. Older siblings are often used to caring for their little brother or sister in some way, and can expand that role when the younger one is sick. But a younger sibling may feel he or she has no real role to play, exacerbating the feeling of being left out.[2]

It is hard to know how common these problems are, but one study examined children six months after the death of a sibling and found that 36 per cent still showed academic, psychological and social problems.[1]

Children under the age of five may be especially prone to problems, as they find it hard to understand all that is happening. They think their parents' absence is a form of punishment and end up feeling guilty and anxious.[1] However, one study suggests they cope better than people think. Research involving 25 children aged three to five who had a brother or sister with cancer showed they were well adjusted and competent. They were better behaved than the average preschooler. Family were extremely flexible and able to adjust to circumstances. In all, it was a favourable picture.[3]

Death

Children react in a wide variety of ways to the death of a brother or sister. Some react with calmness and an appropriate sense of grief—others react with guilt, anxiety, fear of death, loss of appetite, fear of separation from parents and disordered concepts of hospitals, doctors, illness, death and religion.

It is likely that children adapt better if their brother or sister has died at home, rather than at the hospital or hospice.[4] Children whose sibling died at home said they were prepared for it and knew what was likely to happen. Children whose sibling died in a hospital said they were unprepared, felt useless, and isolated from both their parents and their brother or sister.

What to do

Keep an eye on your other children. Watch how they are eating, sleeping and behaving. See if their mood changes.

Respond to any changes you see by asking if there are any worries. Be specific and lead the conversation. Do you know what is happening to your sister? Are you scared he is going to die? Do you think she will get better? Is there anything in particular that is worrying you?

Better still, lead these conversations regularly, and don't wait for problems to appear. Stay open and honest with all your children and keep them all involved. There is a good chance they are experiencing all the fears and anxieties you are feeling.

Involve all your children in their sibling's illness as much as possible. Encourage them to visit the hospital, to ask questions, to make presents for their sick brother or sister, to feel at home in the hospital, to have time to talk to their brother or sister alone without you there.

Encourage all your children to keep up their interests—get them to bring their friends home, to keep up their swimming, or netball, or cricket. or drawing. Allow them to visit their friends.

Take all your children out for special treats. Give each a little time on their own, even if it's only a walk around the block or lunch in the park at times when things are very busy.

Stay interested in them. Ask about their day at school, their friends, their exams, their achievements at sport. Try not to miss tuckshop and sports days, if that's what you did before. Try to change your involvement in their lives as little as possible.

Tell the teachers of all your children about your child's cancer. Make sure they understand that there will be some disruption, but that it should be kept to as little as possible.

If a brother or sister is obviously suffering, and your attempts at help are unsuccessful, then don't wait. Seek professional help.

Coping Styles

Cancer in children, teenagers and young adults is cruel. The early symptoms can be innocuous and overlooked for a long time; the diagnosis can appear without warning of its severity; the treatment and its side effects can seem more painful than the disease itself. People with cancer must believe that treatments which may make them deathly ill will save their lives.[1]

It takes some effort to cope with all these problems, and everybody has their own way of coping. The child is going to react differently to the parent, the brother, the sister, the aunt, the uncle, the grandparents and the friends. Everybody will find their own way to cope. The difficulty is to pick up those who are not coping so they can be helped.

Another point to consider is that people will cope in different ways at different times of their illness. For example, many children will avoid talking about their cancer and treatment in the early stage of their illness, while becoming more involved and accepting later on.[2] This is using the technique of denial as a way of coping.

To understand cancer properly, it can help to think of it as a chronic illness. Your child may survive the cancer and its treatment, but they will have brought significant changes to your child's life. Your child will never be the same person because of the impact of such a serious illness. The changes will last a lifetime.

But most people adapt to the diagnosis of cancer and its treatment. They come through the experience, although there may be hidden scars. What little research there is suggests that younger children who survive cancer are no more likely than their peers to have depression or do poorly in school. They fit into society just as well as other children.[1] Most children get over the ordeal and get on with their lives as people without cancer would, although the picture may be different for adolescents.

Adolescents

One common way adolescents cope is through denial. According to some psychologists, it is a normal way for teenagers to adapt to the stress of the situation and should not be discouraged.[3]

Teenagers might initially deny their illness to themselves, while apparently (and passively) going along with the treatment offered and the course outlined by doctors and nurses. In that way, it is a stage they will work through. Eventually they will come to accept their illness.

At times of extreme stress, or when they relapse, or when treatment becomes difficult and painful, or when a fellow patient dies, teenagers often revert to denial. As long as this does not interfere with their medical treatment or their relationships with family and hospital staff, it does not matter. With the passage of time, or the relief of the stress, they will usually once again accept their illness.

It is possible to both deny your illness and go along with the treatment. Studies have shown that teenagers focus on day-to-day concrete tasks, rather than the 'big picture' of their illness. As well, the great majority of teenagers with cancer expect to improve, even if they have relapsed.[3]

Teenagers use a variety of other methods to cope with their illness. They may intellectualise it by ignoring their feelings and concentrating on the fine details of their cancer and its treatment; or they regress to an earlier developmental level and leave all the worry and decisions to their parents. There is nothing wrong with any of these methods of coping, although they do highlight how much impact the illness has on a teenager's psychological development.

One common way teenagers cope is to see the cancer and treatment as fighting a battle. They tend to use war imagery. They see the chemotherapy as good soldiers battling the enemy cancer cells. Many teenagers find this imagery helpful.[4]

But there are a number of ways teenagers react that do not help. These include panic, extreme hostility, severe depression, withdrawal, isolation and even attempts at suicide.[3] If your child is behaving in any of these ways, you should seek professional help from a psychologist or psychiatrist. Your hospital will be able to put you in touch with one used to dealing with people with cancer.

You can help your teenage son or daughter to cope in a number of ways. These are:

- Maintain an honest and open relationship. Tell him or her everything that is going on. Don't talk to doctors or nurses behind your child's back. Don't talk over the top of your child.
- Give the teenager a sense of control. At this time of their lives, teenagers are seeking more control. To

suddenly lose their newfound independence because of illness can be a harsh shock. Give your child as many options as possible and let him or her choose what to do. Allow your child to continue to make the choices he or she was making before the cancer arrived—what clothes to wear, whether to go out on the weekend or not, what to have for breakfast. Do not automatically take over as if your 15-year-old son was ten again. Encourage your child to ask questions of the doctors and nurses. Encourage them to find out all they can. Help them when they want help, but do not take over unless you are asked to.

• Respect your child's privacy. Leave the room when your child is being examined, allow him or her time to talk to the doctors and nurses without you listening in. Ask what is going on, but don't press. Accept that while you are affected by this illness, it is not your cancer. It is your child's.

• Encourage your child to keep up his or her interests. It was put very neatly by Michael Carr-Gregg, who survived cancer as a teenager, started CanTeen, and became a psychologist specialising in adolescence and illness. He said: 'Adolescents with cancer are not always ill, but are always teenagers, with a variety of interests, sports and hobbies'.[3] Keeping up with normal activities may make your child feel more normal.

• Encourage your child to keep up with friends. In adolescence, the approval and support of peers can be more important than the support of family. Encourage visitors in hospital, make the effort to let your child's friends know how things are going (as some of them may be too scared or embarrassed to ask) and encourage your child to get out and about at home. The psychological boost of seeing friends and talking about teenage concerns can far outweigh the harm from being tired.

• Encourage your child to talk to other people with

cancer. The feeling that they are the only ones to be going through this can be one of the hardest parts of their illness. Groups like CanTeen, Camp Quality and Camp Challenge (see the following chapter, Teenagers, and also Services) are a great way of getting your son or daughter to realise he or she is not alone. Children who go to camps usually have a good time, make a few friends, receive empathy and understanding, and learn about cancer.[5]

Parents

Parents cope in a variety of ways. One effective way is to seek more information about what is going on. The more you learn, the more you feel you will be able to influence what is happening to your child.

Other parents keep busy. They make cakes, repair the car, scrub the house, weed the garden, visit the hospital whenever possible, write to friends, and make sure they do not have a moment alone to sit and think.

Some talk endlessly to friends, relatives and even complete strangers about minute details of their child's disease and treatment. Others say little apart from answering direct questions about their child's health.

It is impossible to say what works and what does not. Do what feels best.

How children cope with amputation

Children who have amputations or seriously deformed limbs might be expected to face social, as well as physical, difficulties. Very little research has been done on this area, but what has been done suggests the social problems can be overcome. The research found that what is important is not how much of the arm or leg the child has lost, but how well he or she is accepted by friends.

So even though you can't replace a lost or deformed limb, you can encourage your child to have confidence and to mix with his or her friends normally. Various methods can be tried to encourage your child's teachers, friends and relatives to show support. With this help, the main social problems can be overcome.[6]

How children cope with changed body image

Many children being treated for cancer undergo great physical changes. They may put on or lose a lot of weight, they may lose their hair or have mouth ulcers and they may develop skin rashes.

After treatment, they may have an amputation or a permanent disability, they may be infertile or they may have chronic pain.

All these things change the way children and teenagers look at themselves, and at their own bodies. They affect their body image. They act as constant reminders that they are different.

It is possible that children with permanent disabilities or deformities will lose some self-esteem. It is possible, although not at all certain, that they may lose self-confidence, withdraw from their friends and become scared of going to school. It may be difficult for them to readjust to normal life.[7]

On the other hand, several studies have shown that people who have amputations before the age of sixteen, and who received extensive rehabilitation and assistance at the time, were just as likely as others to marry, attend university and be employed in good jobs.[8] As far as we can tell, they have normal lives.

After treatment is over

Most of your child's side effects should go fairly soon, although some stay around for a couple of months. Some may last forever.

Some people feel worried or depressed when their treatment is over and they have time to realise what's happened to them. And once the treatment ends, your child will not see the doctors as often. So it may seem as though no-one is looking after your child. The relief that treatment is over is mixed with concern over what happens next.

Remember that your child will go back to the doctor or hospital for follow-up checks. Initially, these may be every three months, then every six months, then every year. Many children's hospitals have adopted the policy of seeing the children who survive cancer every year or two for the rest of their lives. These are called late effects clinics. They recognise that children who survive cancer have particular medical, and sometimes psychological, problems that they need to keep an eye on.

Also, sometimes family members find it hard to continue offering the same level of support as they had shown earlier. The child with cancer can feel, quite rightly, that the support he or she relied on is fading.

Many people who survive cancer feel very angry. They store up feelings about everything that happened during treatment, and have to deal with them after treatment is over. This anger may be at doctors who did not diagnose the cancer earlier, at hospital staff who they saw as rude or impatient or uncaring, at specialists who did not communicate clearly, or at anything and anybody involved. It is often difficult to know how to deal with this anger, but talking about it is a good start.

Others find it hard to give up the 'sick role'. For a year or two or three they have been looked after, driven all over town, the centre of attention. Suddenly that ends.

Even though they regain their health, they find it hard to regain their image of themselves as healthy. They feel like they are still ill, and expect to be treated that way.[9] Changing that behaviour, 'unlearning' it, is not easy. It is not likely to happen by itself. Your child will have to work at it, and you will have to help by talking about your changed expectations of his or her behaviour.

Hypochondria/counterphobia

These words are opposite sides of the same basic problem—the care we take over our bodies. All of us exhibit some basic respect for our bodies. We wash them and feed them. Some people exercise them and stick to healthy diets.

After cancer, it is possible to turn into a hypochondriac. Understandably, every ache or pain or twitch or sniffle can seem as though it is the cancer coming back. Of course it is not, but it is difficult to know that at the time. The hypochondriac cancer survivor gives his or her body almost too much respect. He or she knows what might happen, and wants desperately to prevent it.

But some people go the other way and develop what is called counterphobia. They couldn't care less what happened to them. They drive fast, go hang-gliding, parachuting, often drink too much and take drugs, and generally participate in every risky activity going. Their attitude is this: 'I've faced death and beaten it. Nothing can scare me again.'

With time, people who go either way drift back towards the normal attitude of taking a few risks, having a few worries, but not overdoing either. However, their attitude to life is never the same again.[10]

Summary

There is no one way to deal with cancer. Studies that have looked at the effect of different approaches find that some who embrace their cancer and become experts do just as well as those who try to ignore it. Some people who become argumentative and aggressive towards hospital staff do just as well as those who become passive and compliant. Some take part in everything a hospital has to offer, while others avoid the place like the plague. There is no right or wrong way to approach cancer[1] although there are some ways that are easier for other people to deal with.

Keep a close eye out for any potential problems. Parents often say their children are coping remarkably well with their cancer. Some researchers think this is because the child's distress did not seem to last too long. But they say that because of the rapid development during childhood, even a brief period of turmoil can have long-lasting effects on development.[3] It is important to pick up early any signs that your child is having difficulties.

Teenagers

There is no good time to be told you have a fatal or potentially fatal illness. But to be told your future may be limited at the exact time you are going through that enormous change from child to adult, when you are just recognising you have a future independent of your parents and family, must be a tremendous shock.

Teenagers are at a stage where they are moving towards economic, physical and emotional independence from their family; moving towards understanding their sexuality; establishing a firm set of morals and values; planning a career; and watching and accepting the marked physical and emotional changes they are going through.[1]

One way of looking at adolescence is to see it as a process involving gradual development of four main tasks.[2] These are:
- consolidation of a realistic, stable, positive, adult self-identity—a sense of being comfortable with one's own body;
- achievement of autonomy, especially from parents;

- developing individual sexuality;
- finding a vocation.

How a teenager copes with the diagnosis of cancer depends on a million different things. These include the exact diagnosis, the site of the cancer, treatment offered, likelihood of cure, strengths and weaknesses of the teenager and the social support available.[1]

Often a teenager and his or her family will go through a time of grief, as if death has already occurred. Anger, depression, despair are often what is shown; fear and anxiety are behind it all. What will happen? Will I die? Why me? It's so unfair. These are all normal reactions.

Eventually you all adapt to the situation and start to get on with treatment. Even later, you may accept the situation. But it is fairly common for families to regress to anger and depression and anxiety if treatment is unsuccessful and death looms.

Teenagers have a higher chance than either adults or children of suffering psychological problems from cancer.[3] They are more demanding than either adults or children, and they often recognise this. But the main thing they demand, and respond to, is the presence, understanding, support and company of other teenagers—both their friends and other teenagers with cancer.

Professional support services have always lagged behind the technology. Our arrangement has been described as twenty-first-century technology supported by nineteenth-century psychology. The approach seemed to be that once the body started to respond to treatment, the mind would follow. Help was only offered when severe emotional or behavioural problems surfaced.[4]

In one study, 70 per cent of teenagers said they had problems with their friends and peers after they learnt they had cancer.[5] Many teenagers, like many adults, think cancer is contagious. So these teenagers, at a time in their lives when they most needed help and support, were ostracised and stigmatised out of fear and stupidity.

Such problems only add to a teenager's sense of isolation. Many teenagers already feel that nobody understands them and that they are alone in the world; having cancer makes them feel even more different than they did before.

Teenagers also find it hard to get information about what is going on from their doctors, nurses and families. One cause of this is that some doctors are fairly poor at giving out information. Another is that the teenagers want to be treated as adults and fully informed about everything that is going on, but are too often treated like children. It is important that if you are giving information to your teenager, you repeat it in different ways at different times so he or she understands. Too much information early in a disease can be hard to pick up.

A third of teenagers who have recovered from cancer say they live in fear of relapse and have nobody with whom they can share their fears and anxieties.[6] They are also concerned about their change in appearance, parents' overprotectiveness, loss of control, feelings of guilt and difficulties in leading a 'normal' life.[4]

Particular problems faced by teenagers can be divided into two groups—the social and the psychological.[7] Social problems include:

• rejection by peers, partly due to fears that cancer is catching and the teenager's changed appearance
• disruption to the family
• overprotective parents
• interruption to schooling and career plans.

Psychological problems include:

• fear of going to school
• regression to a younger age psychologically
• failure to comply with medical directions
• denial of illness or need for treatment

• severe anxiety
• behaviour problems
• depression.

The teenager in hospital

Teenagers with cancer have a particular problem when it comes to hospitals. They are not adults, nor are they children. But they must receive treatment in either an adults' hospital or a children's hospital, by an adults' doctor or by a children's doctor. They will be cared for by either an adults' nurse or by a children's nurse. In either case they will feel out of place. Some hospitals and cancer centres have responded to this by developing special adolescent units or wards—others have ignored the problem and hoped it would go away.

The restrictive routine of a hospital ward encourages teenagers to become dependent again. They put the hospital and doctors in control. They force teenagers to become passive recipients of painful and sometimes frightening treatments—anger and fear may be the teenager's (hidden) response. Outpatient care is much preferable, with far less disruption to a teenager's education and social life.[2]

Treatment can also be quite toxic, making the teenager weak, vulnerable and dependent. If they are receiving chemotherapy, they may be prone to infection and may need to avoid their normal social situations.

Body image

At a time when teenagers are coming to terms with their body and the changes it is going through, the treatment and its toxic side effect can be tremendously disruptive.

They may suffer baldness, rapid weight loss or weight

gain, dermatitis from radiotherapy and surgery, or asymmetrical or stunted growth.[2] The shame, embarrassment and isolation they feel can lead them to refuse to go to school, to avoid their friends, to drop out of all social contact.

What teenagers say

CanTeen, an organisation started and run by teenage survivors of cancer, has made a video for teenagers with cancer called 'Been there, done that'. Teenagers talking on the video provide a powerful message. Some selected quotes follow.

When you're first told, the first thing you hear, I think the only thing I heard, was cancer. You don't hear much else, you just hear cancer, and you think—great.

The doctor told me, and I had to be strong, I couldn't cry in front of the doctor. But the minute she left the whole family cried together.

I had a feeling of loneliness that nobody was going to care for me or anything. I really didn't know what was going to happen. I was really scared.

Get your doctor on side and tell him straight that you want to know everything. Even though you're adolescent you've got to make him treat you like an adult, so make sure you're told things and not just your parents, or anybody else. Otherwise you just won't get told things.

You have to remember that's it's your body, and it's not your doctor's body, and it's not your mother's body. You're the boss of your body.

You grow up very quickly. You're faced with all these adult terms and these really harsh treatments . . . and your friends are on the outside. There's really no way they can understand what's happening to you. You're growing, but they're still staying where they are.

The thing that you learn to do is to tell them exactly what's going on. You just turn around and in a calm casual voice you say hey look mate, I've got cancer and I've lost my hair through treatment. It's going to be a pretty hard person that's going to keep up the stirring through that.

When I got sick my mum was really, really overprotective. It wasn't until about seven months later that she'd even let me stay over at my cousin's place. But I can't blame her, because she nearly lost me, and she was just starting to get over it herself.

There's none of this you're a man, you can't cry bullshit. You've got to cry because if you don't it just builds up, builds up, builds up. You can talk, you can talk and talk and talk, but you've still got to cry. The worst thing, I think, that could happen to a person is that they forget how to cry, because when they forget how to cry they lose emotion. That's a really scary thing, and that happened to me once. I just couldn't cry, no matter how hard I tried, then one day it just spilled out and I cried for half a day. I was buggered after that, but Jesus I felt good. You have to accept the fact that you have cancer, and everyone in the family has to accept that you have cancer, and that's the first step to getting better.

Long-term Effects

It is difficult to assess the long-term effects of cancer on a young person. What is it going to mean, when you are forty, to have had cancer at the age of six? This question is becoming more important. At the moment, about one in 600 children develops cancer and about one in 1000 adults have survived cancer as a child. These numbers are bound to increase as the number of children who survive cancer increases dramatically.

Of course, it is difficult to decide when your child has 'survived' cancer. At what stage is your child 'cured'? When treatment is over? Five years after the cancer was first found? It may be wise to look at it this way:

> There is no moment of cure but rather an evolution from the phase of extended survival into a period when the activity of the disease or the likelihood of its return is sufficiently small that the cancer can now be considered to be permanently arrested.[1]

In other words, there is no sudden moment of change, but a gradual shift from treatment towards cure.

What does it mean to be cured? Will having had cancer make a difference to the rest of your child's life? Will the treatment?

A group of American doctors decided to find out by studying all those children who were diagnosed with cancer between 1945 and 1975, and who were treated successfully at hospitals in Los Angeles and Boston.[2] They could find 219 who were still alive and were willing to be interviewed.

Compared with people of similar age, sex and background, people who survived cancer as a child did as well as anybody else at getting through high school and going on to university. They were as likely as anyone else to have steady jobs and incomes were average. They had received some discrimination from the armed services— finding it difficult to enlist—but otherwise faced few problems concerned with work.

One area in which people who had survived cancer faced difficulties was in obtaining life and medical insurance. Health insurance is very important in the United States, because Americans do not have a national health insurance scheme like Medicare. It is hard to know whether these findings are relevant to Australia or not.

The only exception to this generally favourable outcome was people with brain tumours. They faced difficulties finishing school, going to university and getting jobs. Presumably, the damaging effects of surgery and radiotherapy to the brain played a part in their problems.

One point that came from this study was that, compared to people of similar backgrounds, survivors of cancer were more conservative in their outlook at work. They were cooperative, were infrequently disciplined, and rarely requested special provisions in the workplace. They were less likely than average to accept a promotion or move, even when it was deserved. Basically, they were more accepting of their lot and less willing to change.

In another study, three researchers from the US National Cancer Institute followed up 29 people who had survived Ewing's sarcoma for at least five years.[3] These people had all been treated as children before 1974, and were now adults. They wanted to find out how the cancer had affected their lives—not just their health but their work, their chances of marriage, their psychological well-being. They compared the survivors, as they called them, to their brothers and sisters.

All survivors of Ewing's sarcoma said their health was either good or excellent. They were no more likely than the average person to have high blood pressure, heart disease, arthritis, kidney disease, diabetes, problems with sight or hearing, hormonal problems or emotional problems.

They were just as likely as their brothers and sisters to have married and had children.

People who had survived Ewing's sarcoma were more likely to have a physical disability, whether it be from the surgery or radiotherapy. They found it hard to climb stairs, and needed help to drive a car. But they were just as likely to have jobs, and they earned the same income as people who had not had cancer as a child.

The only major difference was that two of the group who survived Ewing's later developed a second cancer.

This study reassures us that surviving childhood cancer does not seem to have a life-long psychological or emotional impact. But there are two shortcomings that mean the study should be treated with caution.

The first is that it compared children with cancer with their brothers and sisters. And as discussed in the chapter, Brothers and Sisters, siblings of children with cancer have their own problems.

The second shortcoming is that these survivors were treated when treatment was milder. Doctors now use stronger drugs and more radical surgery, meaning that the physical impact of treatment is likely to be more severe. On the other hand, children's hospitals now take a much greater interest in the psychological welfare of their patients, so it is possible that these two will balance out.

Young children

Two American researchers interviewed more than 100 school-age children who had survived cancer, and their parents, to see what they thought of the whole experience.[4]

Of the children, 40 per cent had a positive attitude towards their cancer. They said they were glad it was over, or they were lucky to have survived, or they had learnt a lot, or they were better people for it.

The rest had a negative attitude. They were angry, or lonely, or worried about school, or worried about any physical impairments, or their health. Some were concerned that it had strained their parents' relationship. Others said they felt different, without being able to say why.

Cancer in children aged 10–15

Doctors from the University of Pennsylvania decided to study 35 children who developed cancer when aged 10–15, because of the particular changes children go through in this period.[5]

They found that on the whole, these children did well. Psychologically and socially, they varied little from children of similar ages. But a few points of interest still arise.

As time went on, the children who had survived cancer started to feel a little isolated. Perhaps their parents had been overprotective, perhaps they had been away from their friends for too long, perhaps they missed the contact with the hospital and doctors and nurses.

In some ways, it is easier to have cancer as an infant or toddler than as a child or teenager. Schoolchildren are desperate to be accepted by their peers, and time away from school (as well as the fact of cancer and possibly baldness) makes that difficult. As well, changing schools is difficult because children then have to go through the whole process of earning acceptance from their peers. That is difficult when they feel different and vulnerable.

Work

People who have survived cancer may be discriminated against in their search for work because of society's ignorance about cancer. A few examples are:[6]

- High school student cured of Hodgkin's disease, but with chronic pain, met with a vocational guidance counsellor who tried to steer the girl away from a career in nursing because of his misconceptions about cancer and cures. He talked about her need to avoid infection and suggested she would find it hard to get a job.
- Young man who had his leg amputated because of osteogenic sarcoma had been off treatment for seven years. He trained as a cardiac technician, but could not get a job.
- A 15-year-old boy was cured of leukaemia. Four years later, despite his best efforts, he did not yet have a job.
- Young man who had recovered from Hodgkin's disease tried to join the police force. Despite months of appeals and letters from doctors, the police only admitted him after he took legal action.
- Young girl applied repeatedly to enter nursing training, but only gained admission after the hospital board supported her.

There are three main reasons for this discrimination. Some people think that:

- cancer is a death sentence
- cancer is contagious
- people who survive cancer are unlikely to ever be healthy and productive again.

But on the whole, once people who have survived cancer overcome that discrimination and find work, they do it well. Apart from a physical disability which may bar them from heavy or extremely physical work, people who have survived cancer work as well as anybody else.

One study from the US looked closely at how people who had developed cancer as adolescents handled work.[7] The results were very promising. On average, those who had survived cancer in their adolescence earned higher incomes, worried less about their work and were just as likely to have jobs as others. The only worry was that some had been rejected for jobs they thought they deserved. They felt this was due to their history of cancer and the employers' lack of understanding of it.

Other studies have examined what happens to people who are employed at the time they get cancer. Generally, they have shown that 75–80 per cent of those people return to normal work after treatment.[8]

Marriage

Several American doctors and psychologists have tried to work out whether having cancer as a child or teenager alters your chances of getting married. They want to know, because getting married and having children reflect two things—a degree of acceptance by society and an acceptance by the survivor of cancer that he or she has a future.

One study says that men who have had cancer as a child or teenager are less likely than average to marry as adults, although there is no difference for women.[9] When you look at the report closely, it is clear that if you have a brain tumour as a child, you are less likely than average to marry. This is especially true if you have the brain tumour when you are very young. Presumably, this is due to the damaging effects of surgery and radiotherapy on the brain. But if you have any other sort of cancer as a child or teenager, then your chances of marrying as an adult are the same as anyone else's.

Other studies have suggested that people who survived cancer as a child or teenager are less likely to marry,[10] partly because of any physical disabilities as a result of the treatment, but the sex difference is reversed. Men with disabilities marry just as often as men without disabilities. But women with disabilities are less likely to marry, presumably because they do not measure up to society's idealised image of feminine beauty.[11]

But whether or not having cancer does reduce chances of marriage, it has an impact in another way—it makes people feel they are unlikely to be able to marry. They are worried about their fertility, about talking about cancer, and about whether anybody would want to marry someone who had been through such a serious illness.[12]

Flashbacks

One rarely mentioned effect of surviving cancer is that of the flashback.[8] Your child, especially if a teenager or older when diagnosed, may vividly remember the day he or she was diagnosed, or discovered the lump, or started chemotherapy, or had surgery. On that day each year your child may experience all the fear and anxiety that he or she felt. There can even be a feeling of rising tension for a few days or weeks leading up to anniversary. These flashbacks can be very hard to deal with, and they may last many years. Fortunately they are rarely severe, and they usually fade with time.

Guilt

Another rarely discussed problem is what is known as survivor guilt.[8] It is similar to the feelings of survivors of Nazi concentration camps. They feel pleased to be alive, but constantly guilty that they survived while others died.

Of course, the feeling is not as intense in people who survived cancer as those who survived death camps, but it can be a problem that is hard to deal with.

Sexuality and Relationships

The issue of sexuality is vitally important, even when dealing with toddlers. For the toddler will one day be a young woman or man who will go through the same question as the 20-year-old with cancer—can I have a normal sex life? How has the cancer affected me?

What is a normal sex life?

A normal sex life is whatever a person thinks is a normal sex life. It is normal for some people to have intercourse every day, while once a month is normal for others. It is normal for one person to masturbate regularly, while others never do it. It is normal for some people to have oral sex regularly, while others would never dream of it.

But sex is not all there is to relationships. Sex is just part of the human need for closeness—for touching, for cuddling, for play, for closeness. It is possible to have a normal loving relationship without having intercourse or any other form of sexual expression.

What effect does cancer have?

It is normal for somebody with cancer to lose interest in sex. After all, your son or daughter might be feeling quite ill, and might be having treatments such as surgery, radiotherapy or chemotherapy. Those can be enough to make anybody lose interest in sex.

On top of that, there are all the problems that the diagnosis of cancer can bring. Some people with cancer feel quite scared, which makes them lose interest in sex. Others feel dirty or impure. All these feelings are quite natural, even if they are not necessarily accurate.

Sometimes the cancer, because of its location or the treatment required, can cause particular problems. For example, many women who have radiotherapy to the pelvis find intercourse painful because their vagina has contracted. They may also be susceptible to developing vaginal thrush. Or a man who has had radiotherapy to the groin may have some pain in his testicles, which impairs his sexual desires.

But even if cancer or its treatment does turn a teenager or adult off sex, it does not necessarily turn them off the closeness and cuddling and touching that is part of our relationships. It is important to keep this touching and cuddling and closeness going.

Once the cancer is gone

You should find that once the cancer is under control, and treatments are easing up or have finished, sexual needs and desires slowly return to normal.

But it still may prove difficult for the person who has had cancer to express those needs. He or she may feel very self-conscious about scarring, or about an amputated limb, or about an uneven spine, or about the loss of body hair caused by chemotherapy or radiotherapy.

This self-consciousness is particularly common if it involves treatment to the head and neck, the sexual organs or the breast.[1] But any surgery can have an impact on body image, which reflects on feelings of sexuality.

As well, it may prove difficult for the person who has had cancer to relax sufficiently to enjoy sex. Somebody scared the cancer may return is likely to be subconsciously watching their body for signs of cancer. Masters and Johnson have shown that when healthy people monitor their reactions during sex, they get less aroused and sexual problems may occur. If someone who survived cancer is constantly watching themselves, then sex could become a problem.[1]

Other problems could arise from any financial difficulties, marital discord or changes in occupation induced by cancer.

Research has shown that adolescents who have cancer or who have survived it are less likely than other adolescents to form romantic or sexual relationships. Some feel self-conscious about their cancer and find it difficult to believe that anybody would be interested in them.

Some say they want to concentrate on their studies, some worry about whether they will be able to perform sexually, some worry whether they might be sterile, and if they are why bother with sex?[2]

But they rarely express these feelings openly. They are more likely to delay having to confront their sexuality or fertility by not asking about it, by avoiding sexual relationships or by throwing themselves into other activities such as sport, study or career.

What if my daughter has early menopause?

Some women having chemotherapy or radiotherapy to the pelvis for cancer will have an early menopause. Their

ovaries will stop working—they will not produce the female hormones oestrogen and progesterone. This will have quite a few effects on the woman's body, including:
• hot flushes
• mood swings
• a dry vagina
• tendency to osteoporosis (brittle bones)
• infertility.
Several things can be done to help. For a start, she can see an endocrinologist, who is a specialist in hormone disorders, to discuss the need for hormone replacement therapy. Women who have passed menopause can take, as tablets, the hormones their bodies normally make.

Many people worry that an early menopause will interfere with a woman's sexuality. If handled correctly, it should not. Hormone replacement therapy should ease the vaginal dryness that can be mistaken for a lack of sexual desire.

The lack of female hormones does not inhibit desire. Many people think high levels of oestrogen and progesterone make a woman desire sex. But in fact the physical basis of sexual desire largely comes from the small amounts of the male hormone testosterone circulating in a woman's bloodstream. And testosterone is not made in the ovaries, but in the adrenal glands, which sit on top of the kidneys. So even premature menopause should not really affect a woman's sexual desires.[3]

My
Child is
Dying

What does my child understand?

Children understand death differently at different ages. Below is a general guide as to what your child might understand, although it must be stressed that these ages are rough guides only. The more mature child will understand death earlier, as will the child with more personal experience of death in the family.

Somewhere between the ages of eighteen months and three years, children start to develop some concept of death, but it is not the same as ours. They notice that dead things disappear, although they are not sure where they go. They think death is only temporary. They think dead people just live somewhere else and are capable of eating, sleeping, breathing, talking and carrying on a normal life. Just somewhere else.

Around the age of five or six, this concept changes. The child realises that death is permanent, but thinks it can only happen to older people. By the age of eight or ten, the child sees death as final, permanent and

44

irreversible. It can happen to anybody of any age. However most children, and adolescents, and young adults, and middle-aged adults, and some older people, think it is unlikely to happen to them.[1]

Eventually, some time between the ages of fifteen and 150, people come to accept that death is universal, irreversible and permanent.

Stages of dying

The writer Elizabeth Kubler-Ross described five stages of dying. These are:[2]
• denial and isolation
• anger
• bargaining
• depression
• acceptance.
At times these have been held to be rigid stages through which all must pass. In reality, they are stages which people can enter and leave at will. On receiving a diagnosis of cancer, or being told they are likely to die, people can go straight to depression, or acceptance, or anger. They may move around, backwards and forwards, and may even die angry after having accepted their death for much of their illness. But understanding the stages does make it easier to grasp what is going on in the mind of someone who is dying.

Talking about dying

Children and teenagers have a great need to look at death openly. Their concerns focus not so much on the philosophical questions—'is there a heaven?' or 'what is the meaning of life?'—but on simple mechanical aspects of death—'will I die at home?', 'will I be in pain?' and 'will I choke to death?'[3]

So it is important that lines of communication between all members of the family stay open. Everybody should be willing and able to talk to the dying person and answer, as honestly and openly as possible, whatever questions are asked.

Often as a child nears death, members of the family stop communicating with each other and more or less wait for the event. They concentrate so much on the dying child they leave little time and love for each other. This can be quite harmful, as it slows the return back to a more normal family life.[4]

Terminally ill children often choose one person, either inside or outside the family, to talk to.[4] That person will hear more of the child's hopes and fears than all the others put together. It is important for the chosen person to be prepared, to look for signs that the child or teenager wants to talk, and to be open and honest about what is happening. The child or teenager who is dying may only offer one opening to talk—if that opening is neglected then it may be too late.

Many parents want to avoid using words like death and dying. But it is important to use these words, because using other words can be terribly confusing.

For example, parents may tell a child whose sister has died that 'God has taken Mary to heaven because he loves her so much'. The surviving child can become angry, wondering why God loves Mary more than God loves him. Or the surviving child might begin behaving badly, hoping God will love him less.[1]

Also, telling a child that someone else has 'gone to sleep' or been 'lost' may make the child worry about going to sleep or getting lost.

Where should my child die?

Most deaths from cancer are predictable. If your child is dying, it is likely you will know about it days, weeks or even months in advance. That gives you the opportunity to plan a few of the circumstances surrounding your child's death. It also gives you the chance to prepare yourself for it.

Until early this century, everybody died at home. Death was a part of life, especially when families were large and childhood illnesses common and less treatable. It was a rare person who had not had a brother, sister or cousin die as a child.

Improvements in medical care and the growth of hospitals caused a change, so that most people with cancer died in hospital. But now there has been another change, and many hospitals are encouraging people with cancer to go home to die.

The advantages of dying at home are these:
• Family and friends feel comfortable that they can be with the dying child at any time, day or night.
• The child is in his or her usual environment.
• The entire family, especially any other children, can see that what happens is natural.
• It is easier to make sure that you or somebody else is actually there with your child at the moment when he or she dies. Some parents find it very distressing to think their child died alone in hospital, even if they had been with their family almost every minute of the last few months.

The advantages of dying in a hospital or hospice are these:
• The child (or you) may feel safer in a hospital, knowing that expert medical attention is nearby.
• The physical work of nursing the child or adolescent may be too difficult.
• You can usually stay around the clock.

• You can devote yourself to your child's last days or
  weeks without the worry of what else is going on around
  your home.
It is important that, if your child is dying, you and your
child decide to do what suits you. Doctors and nurses
all have their own beliefs about what may suit, but they
don't know you as well as you know yourself. So decide
what you would like to do, and do it. If that option
doesn't work, you can always change and try the other
way.

Brothers and sisters

If your child dies, your other children will react
differently from you, even though you can be sure their
feelings are basically similar. Children under five, in
particular, may seem to behave strangely and appear
uncaring.[1] They may carry on as if nothing has happened,
but this is really their equivalent of an adult's shock and
denial. Or they may take their dead sibling's belongings
away. This is not greed, but their attempt to keep the
dead child 'alive' and nearby.

You should involve all your children with their sibling's
dying, and death. Almost all who work with children
suggest that children should be allowed, or even
encouraged, to attend whatever funeral or remembrance
services are held.

Afterwards

Whole books have been written about dealing with life
after the death of your child. This is not the time and
place to go into detail—if that is to happen it is some
time away. For this book, it may be worth quoting one
parent interviewed for a psychological study:[5]

After a while, you are able to live life again, but never at the same level. There is always that void, that constant pain somewhere deep in the back of your mind, that keeps you from ever being as happy again as you once were.

Fears and Feelings

The cancer stereotype

The cancer stereotype is a particular image—it is what adults expect to see when they see a child with cancer. The child is young, probably bald, and vulnerable; needs a lot of help, becomes sick easily and is incapable of behaving as a healthy child of the same age. You can not expect as much of a child with cancer.

People think children with cancer, even in remission, are less clear-headed, less intelligent, less active, poorly behaved, weaker, less mature and less likely to adjust well in the future.

The labels are false. Children with cancer in remission are just children. They are no less active or intelligent or sociable. It is just that adults think they are. What is worrying is that a self-fulfilling prophecy might occur.[1]

Self-fulfilling prophecies happen through life. We think we are going to pass an exam, so we study hard, absorb the information and pass. We think we are going to have a bad day at work, so we mope around, working little, attract the attention of the boss and get abused. Confidence attracts success, lack of confidence attracts failure.

If children are treated as if they are weak and unintelligent and inactive and poorly behaved, there is always the possibility that they will become weak and unintelligent and inactive and poorly behaved. It is for this reason that the cancer stereotype is so destructive.

The stigma

Most people believe in the notion of a 'just world'. They believe that people generally get what they deserve. In the long run, good things happen to good people and bad things happen to bad people. So when something bad occurs, they tend to blame people's behaviour. You hear it all the time when rape is discussed: 'she shouldn't have been out at night', or 'why was she wearing such a short skirt, anyway?'

It is thought that such comments and 'victim-blaming' do not come from cruelty, but from the belief that we can somehow control our world and what happens to us.[2] We think that if we know what caused a tragic incident, then we can prevent it happening to us.

Unfortunately, many victims accept this explanation. Women who have been raped feel guilty and blame themselves, asking 'what did I do wrong?'

In a similar way, although to a lesser extent, some people blame the person with cancer for their disease. In certain cases where the direct cause is known, this approach may be accurate, even if it is unhelpful. For example, it may be true that someone who smokes heavily is largely responsible for their lung cancer. But it doesn't do any good to say: 'it's all your fault.'

In the great majority of cases though, nobody knows the causes of cancer. This is especially so for cancer in children and teenagers. So blaming the victim is not just rude and demoralising, it is also wrong. Nevertheless, it happens. There are times when people are blamed for getting cancer.

The other side of this is the stigma attached to having cancer. One American researcher tried to highlight this by asking about attitudes to cancer in different ways. People were asked if they would buy a house knowing the previous owner died of cancer. The answer was always 'yes'. But the true attitudes came out when people were asked if they would buy a house knowing the previous owner had died of heart disease. Some of them said: 'yes, it's not like they died of cancer!'[2]

It is worth remembering that people who develop cancer are the same as those who answer questionnaires—so those who have cancer are likely to feel the same way about it as everyone else. They may feel intense shame and self-disgust over their illness. These feelings can be greater in teenagers and younger adults than in older adults.

Fear

Many people who have survived cancer fear that it will come back.[3] They worry that they will die. The worst part is that they have no idea when or how the cancer might come back, so they have no way of controlling their fear.

The good thing is that the fear usually fades with time. People learn to deal with the uncertainty, and most recognise that as time passes the likelihood that the cancer will come back diminishes. But with some people, fear persists for the rest of their lives.

Reactions vary enormously. Some wake in the middle of the night, afraid it will return. Others go as far as contemplating suicide. Some worry constantly about their health.

Survivors of cancer can go a variety of ways over their health. Some end up as hypochondriacs, fearing every ache signals a return of cancer. They go to the doctor with every sniffle and ask for CAT scans to check the cancer hasn't come back. Others avoid doctors altogether, not keeping in touch with their cancer specialists and, when necessary, only seeing doctors who know nothing about their cancer. One explanation is that any contact with the hospital, or doctor, or even waiting room where they spent time during their treatment re-awakens all the old fears. They can avoid the fears by avoiding the doctors and hospitals associated with them.

Schooling

Oddly, school is an important part of cancer treatment. It was recognised two or three decades ago that going to school whenever possible was a crucial part of helping a child recover from cancer. It did not make the child physically any healthier, but it allowed him or her to rejoin normal life, to feel part of the crowd again, to make contact with friends again.

That is not to say that children will find it easy to go to school. They may find it hard to deal with looking different. Or they may be scared that they have missed so much work they will fail. Or they may be worried their friends will have forgotten them, especially if they have been away for a couple of months. Younger children may not want to be separated from their mother.

These difficulties can be compounded by teachers; they are ordinary people who have the same misconceptions about cancer as many other people do. For this reason, some state cancer councils and health departments will make visits to schools to talk about cancer. They make sure the other children are aware of what it means, and what the child with cancer can and can not do, and explain that it is not contagious. They also make sure the teachers understand as much as possible about cancer, so they can make it easier for the child with cancer to stay at school during treatment.

Talking about cancer

Talking to people with cancer can be difficult. It is hard to know what to say, especially when you are unsure of how you feel yourself.

Doctors used to have the attitude that informing people directly that they had cancer was too distressing. Most people cottoned on—they were surrounded by serious-faced people, they had radiotherapy or chemotherapy, and they may even have been treated in a recognisable cancer ward. But the doctors felt that as long as the word cancer was not mentioned, people could keep their illusions.

Then in the 1970s the opposite view was put with more force. This view said that people with cancer and their families were often distressed by the enormous web of deceit between them and tired by the effort of keeping up a pretence. Breaking down those barriers led to a great sense of relief. It was suggested that 'the malignant reputation of cancer is enhanced by the secrecy surrounding it'.[4]

The consensus now seems to be that speaking the truth at all times does more good than harm. Even at a young age, children appear to understand death without necessarily fearing it. And even if they don't understand death, they have enough insight to register that the future is uncertain.[5] However if adults give the impression that death can not be discussed, that heightens anxiety in the child.[6]

But even if doctors decide to speak the truth, the whole truth and nothing but the truth, it seems the message does not always get through. British doctors interviewed 100 people with cancer and their doctors, to see whether both sides had the same impression of what was going on. They found that one-third of those with metastases thought their cancer had been contained, and one-third of people being treated for pain relief without hope of a cure believed that the drugs would cure them. Yet every doctor said they had given the right information.[7]

As well, most doctors caution against trying to force children and their families to listen to what they don't want to hear. They say that while open and honest communication should be the aim in most cases, some people truly prefer not to be confronted.

Dr Stewart Dunn, a psychologist with Sydney University, decided to see if it made any difference to people with cancer to call it by another name. In a variety of situations, he carried out interviews and questionnaires using either 'cancer' or the general phrase 'illness'.[8]

One of the findings was that if people use the word cancer openly, then the people with cancer feel able to cope with it, even though it does make them more anxious for a short while. But if people don't use the word cancer, then they worry that it is so frightening that it can not even be talked about.

Loneliness

People with cancer often miss out on the emotional and social support they need so much. This occurs for four main reasons:
- Cancer carries a social stigma. People are scared of it, they think it's contagious, they feel helpless when confronted with somebody with cancer.
- Many people find it difficult to talk about cancer. This includes people with cancer, family, friends and medical and nursing staff.

• Friends and family may have ambivalent attitudes towards people with cancer. They are obviously uncomfortable yet they feel they should be cheerful and optimistic. This obvious falseness may make the person with cancer avoid social contact.
• Physical disabilities may prevent people with cancer participating in social activities.[9]

Following from that, it seems obvious that people with cancer might feel lonely. A group of Israeli psychologists and social workers decided to see if this was true. They found, to their surprise, that people with cancer were no more lonely overall than healthy people (although they admit that their study did not include people with serious physical disabilities).

But some interesting things came out of the study. First, people with cancer do feel lonely when they are undergoing treatment—at the hospital or clinic, visiting the doctor and so on. They could do with extra support at those times. Second, unmarried people with cancer feel lonely more often than married people. They may lack the constant support available.

PART 2

Soul—what the people say

Interviews

Diane Bond

Interview with Diane Bond and her parents Jessie and Don in their Sydney home. Diane was born on 7 February 1967, and was 26 at the time of our interview.

Diane I started having cramps in my leg and I was waking up in the middle of the night with a lot of pain. That happened a couple of times I was putting Dencorub on my leg, thinking that would help it because it was just a muscle strain or something.

We were going away to Tasmania fairly soon so we went to the doctor, who did a test on it, then a biopsy, then told us what was going on. So there went Tasmania—we didn't go on our holiday. It was all very quick once I saw the doctor.

Jessie You saw one doctor Thursday, the specialist Friday, you were in hospital Monday and had the biopsy Tuesday.

Mark How long had you had the cramps for?

Diane Not very long. I suppose a week or two before I

went to the doctor. It was only a few nights that it kept me awake for a few hours.

Mark   And how old were you?

Diane   Seventeen. It started in April when I was seventeen and it finished just before my eighteenth birthday the following year.

Jessie   We thought it was just growing pains. But the doctors were very quick.

Mark   So you only had three or four days in that period of thinking it was cancer but not knowing.

Diane   Well I didn't really know then, either. I was very very naive, right the way through. I didn't have a clue what was going on.

Jessie   They said it was a tumour, but nobody really thought it was cancer until they said it was malignant.

Don   But Dr Marsden [the orthopaedic surgeon] did say it looked like it was pretty nasty. That's when she had the biopsy. We were up there and he rang through to the ward and said it didn't look all that good. So we were sort of prepared for whatever might have happened.

Mark   Did somebody actually come and say to you: 'This is cancer. This is what we're planning'?

Diane   They never used the word cancer which, for me, was good. I think hearing the word cancer would have been a bit more alarming. At seventeen I was very naive, and I think it was to my advantage. I never felt that I had anything to worry about, that this was going to kill me. I had a positive attitude the whole way through. I still hated having chemotherapy, but I never felt that this was going to be it.

Mark   What word *did* they use?

Diane   They called it a tumour, which wasn't as scary. They called it a sarcoma a few times, too.

Jessie   Tumour was the word they used most.

Diane   When I was in hospital they didn't call it cancer. I suppose if you take it that step further you know that's what it is.

Mark   Did you have the cancer anywhere else?

Diane   No, it was only in the one spot. Actually, my Mum's niece had exactly the same thing when she was sixteen. She had her leg amputated and died from it. You'd think that would make it click in my head a bit more— hey, this is dangerous. But it didn't. I always thought they'd got to it at a stage where they could cure it.

Jessie   Also, it was a few years ago that she passed on. We thought that things had improved a little since then.

Mark   So what treatment did you have?

Diane   I had chemotherapy—I had six lots of that. Then I had the operation where they took out the fibula [the bone on the outside of the shin]. Then they decided to give me radiotherapy as well, but they also decided because of my age that it was just as well to have another lot of chemotherapy after that to be on the safe side. I wasn't too impressed about that because I thought I'd finished with all that. I found the surgery and the radiotherapy easy, but the chemotherapy . . . just the thought of it.

Jessie   She said she'd rather have more operations and not the chemo.

Diane   Yes, well, a couple of years later I had another operation where they split the tendon to my foot in half.

Mark   How does it all work?

Diane   OK. I wore a splint for about five years, and I've only just stopped wearing it. The doctor said I should still be wearing it, and I might have effects later in my life, but at the moment I'm fine.

Mark   Do you play sport?

Diane   No, I'm not the sporty type. I go out swimming and I've been playing the odd game of tennis in the last few weeks, but I'm not a netballer or a softballer or anything like that.

Mark   So it doesn't slow you down too much?

Diane   No. No. I still can't wear high heeled shoes, and I

find that a bit hard. I suppose if I was desperate I could, but ...

Mark   What was it about the chemo that got you?

Diane   Actually having it. I was all right up to the time, and afterwards it was like a real bad dose of the flu, but waiting for it ... For the first six times I was in hospital overnight. I used to hate it once Mum had to leave, although I knew she had to leave. Just lying there in bed by yourself. The feel of it. You know that it's going to make you sick.

Mark   Did you mind being by yourself at other times?

Diane   I wasn't. I dragged Mum everywhere. That's why I stopped staying overnight. When they started the second lot of chemo, I'd wait the whole day at the hospital trying to get a bed, and finally I'd get a bed at 6 o'clock at night then they'd give me the chemo at 8 o'clock in the morning. You just build up with the nerves. So it was better to come home at night, even though the car trip was pretty bad.

Mark   How long did the treatment last from start to finish?

Diane   April to February. About ten months.

Mark   What was your frame of mind during that time?

Diane   Towards the end I was more realistic about what was going on. I was nearly through it, and I knew they'd given me that extra lot of chemo just as a precaution. I suppose it did get a bit easier towards the end, although I just wanted to get it over and done with. I said I wanted it finished by my eighteenth birthday, so I could start my life afresh.

But of course it doesn't because every three months you've got doctors appointments and blood tests and CT scans—that sort of stuff goes on for months and months afterwards.

Mark   Do you still have regular check-ups?

Diane   Until the year before last I still used to see Dr Kefford, the oncologist who looked after me. Then he said I could start seeing my local GP. I kind of put that off a little bit, but I finally went in December, although I should have gone in February last year.

Dr Marsden? Just recently I stopped going. That was after he told me I'd be wearing the splint for life, so I took the splint off.

Mark Did you like to go back to see them? Were you reassured?

Diane Yes, especially with Dr Kefford because I built up a lot of trust with him. Even when he said I could go to my local GP he said that if I ever had any problems, all I had to do was ring up and he would see me within two weeks. He made it clear that even though he wasn't seeing me regularly, he was still available for me. And I trusted him, too.

Mark How did you find the radiotherapy?

Diane That was a breeze. I had no problems with that, no side effects. I believe some people suffer from nausea, but I didn't notice anything at all.

Mark How did your friends react to the fact that you weren't around so much? To the fact that you had cancer? To the fact that your hair fell out?

Diane See, that was another thing. My hair had finally started to grow back and they gave me the chemotherapy again and I was bald again.

My friends were all fairly good about it. They were good as far as coming to visit me and that sort of stuff. But I think they all understood that sometimes I couldn't be definite about saying yes or no about going out. Also, at seventeen, I couldn't get into pubs anyway, because I looked too young.

Mark Do you have to show your ID now?

Jessie That's one of her sore points.

Diane Even in hospital they'd ask how school was going, and I'd have been working for twelve months.

But socially it didn't affect me too much because it wasn't like I was going out all the time anyway. If anything it was going to the movies and things like that anyway.

It also brought back a friendship. My next door neighbour and I were very good friends until I started high school and we drifted our own way. Then when this happened, we became friends again and have been very good friends since.

Jessie   I think TV has helped a lot, it's made people more aware of what's happening. People can see the results of chemo now, and they understand a bit more about it. And I think the wigs they have now are so good.

Diane   Mind you, I think mine was disgusting.

Jessie   I only had one lady say to me 'Oh, dear, are you going to tell anyone else about it?' as though it should be hush-hush. I say 'Yeah, of course we're going to tell people about it.'

Mark   How about you, Don? Did you find any problems with friends?

Don   Everybody supports you when you're in a community. There were no dramas as far as that was concerned. People naturally are more concerned about what's going to happen than what has happened, and the progression and the treatment, but it's not one of those things that you dwell on. It's part of your life and you get on and live your life as normally as you can.

Mark   Do you have other children?

Diane   Yes, I've got an older sister Christine, who's 28, and a younger brother Peter.

Mark   You said you tried to get on with your life as normally as you could. But there would have been lots of disruptions and trips to hospital and so on. Did you try to go as a family? Did you try to make sure the other two got on with their lives with as little disruption as possible? How did you deal with the family life?

Don   Well, she wasn't away all that much.

Diane   There was the operation, and I was about two

weeks on holidays, I mean in hospital. Then there was overnight a few times.

Don We'd go there, we'd drop her at the hospital in the morning and pick her up of a night time. The old taxi service was part of the deal.

Mark But it wasn't an enormous disruption.

Jessie No, not at all. And living in Sydney helped.

Mark Diane said she never thought she was going to die. Don, Jessie, what did you think?

Don The first thing we thought of was Jessie's niece.

Jessie And when she had the operation, we really didn't believe they wouldn't take the leg off. They said they wouldn't, but you just don't believe it until you see it and know that everything's all right.

Don That was our major fear initially. But the further the treatment went, the greater faith that we had in what was going on.

Mark How long did it take for you to change from worried to hopeful or confident?

Don I don't think we ever lost faith in her.

Mark I'll put it another way. When did you stop being so scared?

Don You never stop being so scared. But it's one of those things that you gradually put behind you. You don't dwell on it. But subconsciously it's always with you.

Mark Still?

Don Oh ... yes and no.

Jessie Well, it's made us appreciate life. If you want to do something, don't put it off. When you've had a close shave, you think a bit differently. You make sure you enjoy life.

There was only one time I pushed the panic button, and that was after the operation. I was coming down the lift and I met one of the sisters, who said: 'We're starting chemo tomorrow.' And I thought: 'They're not telling me everything, they've found another one'. I was really panicking that time. Very much so.

Diane　They all knew about it, and I didn't know about it yet. So my sister was ringing up and pretending that she didn't know anything, and keeping it all cheerful. Because I thought that that was all behind me. It was bad news to me. I found the operation so easy, even though it was quite a major thing, but the chemo ...

Don　He just didn't want to take the risk.

Jessie　But you just doubt what's going on. You don't have enough information to really know for yourself.

Mark　Do you think it's made any difference to you as a person? At seventeen your whole life is changing, then you have this on top.

Diane　I was always a fairly quiet person, so having cancer at that stage didn't help my confidence any. But you get past that. It took a while, I suppose. But I would have been a quiet person anyway, so it's a bit hard to tell whether that made it worse or not.

　　I always found it hard to tell people about it. They'd see me wearing a splint and they'd ask what had happened. For years and years I'd say: 'I had an accident' or: 'I had an operation', but I wouldn't say: 'I had cancer', whereas now I can do that without any worries.

Mark　What was stopping you?

Diane　I don't know. I was worried about the reaction of 'Cancer, you've had cancer'. It didn't seem to, I don't know, I just didn't like it. It just seemed like a bad thing to have. Most people knew, but occasionally you'd get people asking.

　　I suppose I tried to put it behind me by not thinking about having had it, so when I did meet new people I didn't like to dwell on the fact that I'd had it. But now I don't see it as a bad thing any more. If the subject comes up, I'll talk about it.

Jessie　But she went to give blood the other day and they said no, because she'd had it.

Diane　That was eighteen months ago.

Jessie Yes, but it still crops up all the time.

Mark Do you have any particular worries because you have had cancer?

Diane The only aspect is kids. I've been told I've just got to try and see.

Mark So you don't know.

Diane No.

Jessie I thought there'd be a few tests she could have, but they say there's not.

Mark From what I understand, if you don't have periods then you can't, and if you do have periods then there's no way of knowing.

Diane Well, I've kept on regular, although that's something I could happily have got rid of. But it doesn't concern me that because I've had it once it makes it more likely for me to have it again.

Jessie Things have improved a lot. These cancer clubs are fantastic. And when Diane went in, she was too old for the Children's Hospital, so they put her into the old people's ward. They had their teeth out, or they couldn't hear, and she was so young.

Diane At one time I was very depressed because there was this old lady in the bed opposite and she cried for two whole days. This is when I had the operation. She was in a lot of pain.

Jessie But nowadays they've got teenage wards, and they know how to go about it a bit better.

Diane They didn't have CanTeen* going then, and that would have helped.

Mark Do you know there's another one called CanYa? Similar to CanTeen, but for young adults.

Diane No, never heard of it. For people in the same position as me? Or for people who have it now?

Mark For anybody. Basically for people 20 to 35 [see

* CanTeen is a support group for teenagers with cancer. It has offices in each state and territory. (See pages 26–31.)

chapter, Teenagers, and Services, for details]. Do you think the cancer changed your relationships with your parents, and your brother, and your sister?

Diane I was always fairly close to my sister anyway, so I don't think it's changed that at all. I don't think it's changed my relationship with my brother at all. He still treated me the same, and we had our play fights like usual.

Mark You weren't treated as though you were a bit delicate?

Diane I'd always use it as an excuse—watch my leg and so on. Gosh, you've got to use whatever excuse you've got. He's a big boy.

   No, I don't think so. Naturally I spent a lot of time with Mum, because Mum came everywhere with me. And Dad came whenever it was important, so he was there just before the operation, and he'd drive me in, but of course he'd have to go to work, but he'd be there again at night time when I was in hospital, so he'd come and spend some time with me.

Jessie I was lucky that I wasn't working, so I had the time to spend with her. I think that was important.

Diane You're sitting there for hours and hours and hours. Just to have someone sitting there with you is good. And to drive you around—well, I didn't have my licence then anyway.

Mark Were you a young 17 or an old 17?

Diane I was only young.

Mark You didn't have a lot of independence that the cancer made you lose?

Diane No. Even though I'd been working for a while, I was pretty quiet.

Jessie She always went out and did her own thing, but it's just that we're a close family, I suppose. Actually, I thought having to talk to nurses and doctors made her more confident.

Diane Did you? Maybe, but work-wise it didn't.

Mark   What work were you doing at the time?

Diane   I've been working with the National Bank for the last nine years. I was fairly lucky with time off, there was no problem there. But I think it was more around the people I was working with. I was very lucky, I had very understanding bosses.

But after I'd been through it all, that was when I didn't want to go telling everybody what had happened. I just didn't want to have to dwell on it. You're going off to doctors all the time as it is.

[Peter arrived]

Mark   Some people say they miss all the contact with the doctors and hospital. They feel lost. Do you?

Diane   No, because between seeing Dr Marsden, seeing Dr Kefford, having CT scans and blood tests ... Then when that started to ease a bit, I went and had another operation anyway, so no. No. No. Not at all.

Jessie   In fact she started to be a hospital expert.

Diane   I liked Westmead because it didn't have that smell to it—you know that smell hospitals get? I only went to Westmead to see Dr Kefford, not to stay in there.

Jessie   But Prince Alfred, well, Prince Alfred was a very old building and Diane used to get quite confused. They'd say: 'We'll take you off for a test' and the next thing she'd know she's going across Missenden Road into another building. And not expecting it, so she wasn't prepared.

Diane   They asked if I wanted to put a dressing gown on and I said no, because I was warm enough inside, but he didn't say I was going outside. I didn't even put my wig on.

Jessie   It is a public road, and a very busy one. I think it helps if you have a bright clean ward. But the nurses have been fantastic.

Diane   And Dr Kefford was, too. He was great. Right from the word go, from the first day he saw me, he said: 'I think you're going to be OK, you've got the right attitude.' But waiting around in the hospitals all the time for chemo was not much fun.

Mark Did you go to work next day?

Diane No, it would normally be a couple of days before I went back. I tried to get back as soon as possible, and sometimes I probably went back a day too soon, but my boss was very very good. I felt that if I could get back in there, it would take my mind off everything. Sitting around the house was no good.

And with him being so good, it made me want to put myself out a little bit, even though I probably didn't do that much. Getting back to work made it easier.

I went through three stages—I didn't eat and would be throwing up for a few days, then I'd get back into it and eat like crazy, then I'd be sick again.

Don You used to get muscular twitches, too, didn't you.

Diane Yes, that was obviously one of the effects of the drugs I was having.

Jessie I think Peter felt a bit left out by all this. You didn't really know what was going on, did you?

Peter Oh, it was all right. It didn't matter. She had cancer, that's what mattered. You never said she was going to die, so I never worried about it.

Jessie But it was hard on him. He had people ringing up all the time while we were out at the hospital, and he was trying to answer their questions.

Peter I never knew where you were.

Jessie Because all the attention was on Diane.

Diane All those people would be asking how I was, and nobody would be asking how he was.

Jessie But people were very kind. One of our neighbours is an ex-nurse, and she came in and asked if we needed any help with the terminology and she explained it to me. I was really pleased with that information because it does go over your head. They presume you know it.

Diane Even doctors appointments. We found it good to

have the two of us there, because Mum would catch on to something that I'd miss and I'd catch something that she'd miss. We'd discuss it afterwards, because there's just too much to take in straight away.

Also I'd get quite emotional whenever doctors were talking to me about it, so I'd miss half of what they were saying to me anyway. That's probably why I didn't understand things.

At first when they told me what had to happen, I asked Dad and I said: 'What if I don't do it?' And he said: 'They're like your mother's plants. If you don't pull them out straight away, they just grow more and overtake the place.' I thought that was a very good explanation.

Christina Brock

Interview with Christina Brock in her Sydney home. Born 5 January 1960, Christina was aged 33 at the time of interview.

Christina I was diagnosed with Ewing's sarcoma in November 1979. I had presented earlier that year with pains down my right leg. After a couple of months of investigation a biopsy of the joint was done, and it was found I had a Ewing's sarcoma. I had it in my sacroiliac joint in my pelvis, with no metastases in my lung but one in my right tibia. So my primary was inoperable and the metastasis in my leg was never really investigated any further, but it disappeared with treatment.

Mark Between the time the pain started and the time you received a diagnosis, what did you think was going on?

Christina I was told I had sciatica, which is a pretty meaningless term. It just means pain in the leg involving the sciatic nerve. Right up until I was told I had cancer, that wasn't a consideration at all, except just before it was diagnosed. I was to have a biopsy of the joint, and the surgeon came and sat me down and said: 'Sometimes we find things we can't cure.'

He was telling me I had cancer, but I just wasn't receptive at all. I was going home for the weekend and I just wanted to get out. In retrospect, my rheumatologist who had been looking after me hadn't considered cancer at all. She thought I had an infection in my joint. And I think that's basically because you don't expect to get cancer when you're young. So I started chemotherapy and radiotherapy in hospital . . .

Mark   Go back a step. Then they told you that you had cancer. And you were nineteen. What impact did that have?

Christina   I was really sick after the anaesthetic, and I was having some Omnipon to help with the bone pain, and that was making me physically sick as well as the side effects of the anaesthetic.

Mum and Dad decided they wanted to tell me, so they turned off the drip and I came back to the land of the living, but I don't remember them telling me that I had cancer. It was really a gradual realisation over the next couple of days as I had further tests, looking for further metastases in my body. I guess I was in the classical denial stage. Talking to other people, other patients, they have also experienced that sense of unreality. There's also lots and lots happening, so you're really carried along at that stage.

Mark   Because you're part of a routine and a system, you just go with the flow.

Christina   Yes. But Mum and Dad assure me they told me I had cancer and I seemed to understand what they were saying, but I just don't remember being told at all.

Mark   What happened to make you realise it?

Christina I had a really aggressive registrar. I was in a rheumatology ward and they weren't used to cancer patients, let alone nineteen-year-old cancer patients, and the staff were pretty freaked out about that. I think a lot of younger staff members have trouble treating younger cancer patients because they identify with them.

Anyway, I knew how important these other tests were and his inability to understand my need to know the results immediately . . .

I don't know, it was a gradual realisation. It wasn't one event that made me realise I had cancer. However when the oncologist appeared on the ward, this fantastic man who was going to help me, it all became very real when he started to talk about chemotherapy and losing my hair and the possibility of infertility and all that sort of thing. Then I had my next treatment the day after, and I certainly knew what was going on when I had that one.

I can remember looking out the window as this poor young intern tried to find a vein, and there was this fantastic sunset, and I was really very keen to start treatment because it meant I could go home. I'd been in hospital for six weeks by this stage—it wasn't the pain, but the fact that they couldn't diagnose what was going on. They didn't biopsy the joint until I'd been in for four weeks, the other scans were inconclusive. So it was really only at that point that it was diagnosed.

So I remember him being very nervous and missing my vein, and not really understanding why I wanted to get on with the treatment, and him saying 'you won't really want to have this', so I guess I was just carried along with the whole situation. Hospitals are like that—it's like a city within a city, totally cut off from the outside world.

Mark So you started your chemo.

Christina That was pretty horrific. I thought I was fairly

well prepared for what was going to happen—the intensity of the vomiting and the nausea. The staff, not being used to patients being given chemotherapy, were ... OK. The rheumatologist had wanted me to go to the cancer ward to have chemo, but I had begged her to let me stay because I'd wandered around to a phone near the ward and I'd heard somebody vomiting, and it sounded they would vomit forever. I just couldn't bear the thought of going to that place, so I pleaded with her. Hence, when I did have my chemo, the staff were pretty unprepared for it.

Mark   How long did the chemo last?

Christina   I had chemo for nineteen months as an outpatient. It was a really long haul. I had a three-weekly course, which is pretty standard, and they actually still give the same drugs that I had initially. Six months down the track my cancer started to regrow, and that's a fairly common side effect when you have tumour-resistant cells and they become dominant.

So a different line of chemo was decided upon, a cocktail of drugs that was much more aggressive. So I had more neutropaenic episodes* and needed transfusions and platelets and what have you. That was when I would go into hospital and be barrier nursed, which was pretty horrible. I'd get a very low white cell count and get an infection, hence I'd have to be protected from getting more infections.

Mark   Could your friends and family visit you?

Christina   Yes, they did. They all gowned up. Dad used to spend hours and hours with me in hospital. Either Mum or Dad would be with me when I was in hospital, which was nice.

Mark   Did they stay the night?

* A neutropaenic episode is an episode in which Christina's white cells died because of the chemotherapy. It left her extremely vulnerable to infections.

Christina No, but they'd stay until late.

Mark What were the hardest things about chemo to cope with?

Christina After six months of the second regime, I had a really severe neutropaenic episode when we were on holidays up north, and I had to be flown back by air ambulance because I started to fit, and was bleeding from the bowel and all that sort of thing.

At that point, it was just before my twenty-first birthday, I decided I wanted to stop chemo, because I just couldn't see an end in sight. I didn't actively want to die, but I was just tired of living. I think I really needed to meet someone who had been through a similar experience because the isolation and the loneliness were the worst parts of having cancer, just feeling that this had never happened to anyone else. The reality was that you were in a ward of cancer patients, but most of them were quite elderly and that was meaningless, I think.

Mark Were you isolated from your friends?

Christina They were fantastic.

Mark But they didn't have cancer.

Christina No, no. One of my friends actually kept saying to me that he knew what I was going through, so I thought 'OK, why don't you come to the clinic with me when I have a bout of chemotherapy'. He did, and he stayed the day with me, but from that point on he stopped saying he knew what I was going through. It was just horrendous. Towards the end of my treatment my parents almost had to physically drag me to finish off my treatment. They'd come home from work and cajole me to get me into the car. I'd refuse to speak to anyone at the clinic, and was very aggressive and unhappy. I didn't want to be there. It would have been very hard for them to drag me.

Mark Did you tell them you didn't want to go, or did you just passively resist.

Christina I think I was pretty passive-aggressive. The only time I actually told them 'no' was when I stopped treatment for a couple of months.

Mark When did you stop? Was it after that bad episode?

Christina Yes, it was about twelve months down the track.

Mark At that time, did you think you were going to be cured?

Christina I just couldn't see any point to it all. I knew I was going to die if I didn't have more treatment, but I just thought the cure was worse than the disease.

Mark What made you change your mind?

Christina I had a break. Then my oncologist called me and we agreed to remove one drug. I think that consultation, and me feeling empowered, and in control, made me feel better. So we agreed I would have two more courses, and that's what I had. It helped me finish.

But that loss of control was a huge issue for me, and still is. Especially in my medical treatment, I really feel I need to have some say in what's going on, because it's my body. While that sounds very reasonable to anyone who hasn't been sick and who hasn't been through the system, it's actually very hard to have that control.

Mark So if you were going through it again now, what would you do to make sure you had more control?

Christina I'd choose my doctors very carefully. The doctors I see now I have chosen because I like them. Well, I respect them and I think they respect me, too.

Mark How do you go about choosing a doctor?

Christina It's trial and error, and recommendation. If you don't like them, you move on.

Mark What else?

Christina That's hard to answer. I felt I was very well informed, though my oncologist didn't provide any information unless I asked him. But he was always honest with me if I asked him a question.

I think being older, I'm more self-assured now. At that stage I was just becoming independent and gaining that self-assurance from being at uni, and so I would approach my disease . . . I was going to say more rationally but that's not right. I would probably approach it in a more philosophical way, though very willing to give it everything I've got. I'd still fight, but . . . it's a very important question, but I'm finding it hard to answer it.

Mark What were you doing before you got sick?

Christina I was in second year, doing a science degree at Sydney Uni.

Mark What were your plans?

Christina To be a scientist, perhaps a dietitian. I'd always wanted to do science, and I got into it and was enjoying it at uni. I didn't think it was the be-all and end-all, but it was enjoyable. And I was enjoying the social life.

Mark Can you think of ways your cancer has changed your approach to science, your approach to your career, your choice of career?

Christina I went into remission in 1981 but I didn't go back to uni until 1984. I had a couple of attempts before that and just couldn't hack it. Part of the reason was that I felt very isolated and very different. I was older than my peers at uni and just didn't feel that I fitted in, even though the university went out of their way to accommodate me. The two departments I had subjects left in were just fantastic. So it was a huge effort to go back to uni, but I passed. I had to fulfil the requirements that other students did, so while they were understanding I still had to sit my exams and everything. I found it very hard to study because I still had the pain in my leg and was still fairly anorexic from my chemotherapy—that was very much a long-term side effect.

So when I got my degree, it was worth high distinctions even though I got passes, and I felt very

motivated and I really wanted to, well, cure cancer.
Naively. I got a job in immunology because it was the
first one I could get, but I have been very happy being
in that field, and perhaps a bit more aware of who
Nobel Prizes are given to—they're given to people
toward the end of their career for their lifetime of
work, rather than one brilliant discovery, although I
still live in hope that perhaps ... But I'm probably a
bit more realistic about what science is about.

I feel quite driven. That's part of my reasoning for
doing a Master's degree, a yearning for more
knowledge about the immune system and that area of
medical science. Also my cancer has made me quite
impatient, which I don't think is a positive side effect.
That's tied up with being quite driven. But I'm
learning that I'm not going to die tomorrow and that
I have more time, so perhaps in time I'll become more
patient and more methodical. But it's taken me quite
a long time and I'm still quite impatient. It's twelve or
thirteen years since my cancer was diagnosed.

Mark   When did you stop worrying that you were going
to die tomorrow?

Christina   I went into remission in 1981 and I was so-called
'cured' five years later in 1986. Within my family we've
been very conscious of things like that—five years, ten
years and so on. I guess after five years you start to feel
comfortable.

A couple of years ago I had a major scare where I
had what I thought was some metastases in my liver. It
happened very suddenly. I had a routine annual scan,
and it was just after my father had died very suddenly,
so it was a very traumatic time. It brought back a lot of
fear and anxiety, and fear about being a patient again
and losing control, and having to go through the
system again.

Having said all along I would never ever ever have
any more chemotherapy, I would have started the next

day and had whatever it would have taken. I was distraught. I had stupidly read my report, not expecting to find anything but there it was—four lesions on the liver. Conclusion: metastatic liver cancer. I was coming down the lift and just started to cry. I walked back up to the hospital and found my boss and we had a look at the scans together and I've got a friend who's an oncologist and she came and looked at them.

By the time I saw my oncologist I was pretty distraught. I had rung my mother and asked her to come in, never ever having done that before. That was an enormous point of contention between us that I always saw the oncologist on my own. She knew something was up. We spent three very tense days before I could have my liver biopsied, and then it was confirmed that it was not metastatic and it was decided that it was the result of the oestrogen that I was taking as hormone replacement.

But even so, every follow-up scan has caused that apprehension. It's happened before that something unexpected could happen, and reliving those feelings of being a patient again . . . So I think it's always there, but you try to put it into perspective. Every time I get a lump, or a headache, I don't think I've got a brain tumour or anything like that, but it was just that it was so unexpected and I felt so well. Rationally, metastatic liver cancer from a Ewing's cancer is unknown. And it's a pretty unusual spot for a second malignancy, which is more likely at this stage.

My oncologist was very good when we sat down together, very calm, but it was really scary.

When I was doing my Master's qualifying, I had to write four essays and one of them was on a cancer-related area. It was on using monoclonal antibodies in cancer treatment. In doing that I found quite a few articles on Ewing's, and I must admit I started to look them up, and they were all so negative, especially about Ewing's with the primaries being in the pelvis, I didn't ever realise the prognosis was so terrible.

Mark You had it in the pelvis, and you had metastases. If someone was going to tell you your chances, based on the literature, you would have to be told you had a 10 to 20 per cent chance or something like that.

Christina My oncologist always said 75 per cent right from the beginning, but I think that was probably pretty optimistic.

Mark But what did you think your chances were? Do you think it would have made any difference if you thought your chances were much poorer?

Christina In the beginning, I felt I was going to beat it. I'd have a year off uni, and have a bit of treatment, and it would be pretty yucky, but it would be easy. I had absolutely no idea what it would be like, and I'm sure my family had absolutely no idea, either. We had no contact with cancer—no grandparents or relatives or friends who'd had it.

Even when I relapsed, and had the second line of treatment, and that second line had a 20 per cent chance of working, at the time I thought they were really good odds. It's interesting that that reflects how you view a situation and how positive I was feeling at that stage.

Mark I suppose if the alternative is death, then a 20 per cent chance is not bad.

Christina Yes. It's one in five, and I was the one. That was really nice, it was good. But it was really heavy going. Chemotherapy is just horrendous because of the rigmarole you go through. Having drips, and my veins were terrible. At the beginning they were fine and they're just awful now. I have none. It's all a nightmare, really.

The whole procedure became traumatic. It wasn't just the vomiting from the drugs, it was everything.

Mark At the time you were nineteen, and presumably
you had long black curly hair then, too. Did you lose
it?

Christina I was as bald as a badger. It was traumatic when
it was falling out. It started almost immediately, and
Mum said to me once: 'I wish it would all come out in
one go.' Because after a shower there would just be
hair everywhere in the bathroom. But once it was gone,
it was gone. That was fine.

One of my friends actually said to me that I looked
fantastic bald. I didn't wear my scarves if I was at home,
and I hated my wigs so I always wore my scarves. They
were much cooler in summer. I had that adolescent
attitude of trying to shock people by taking my scarves
off in shopping centres.

It's interesting. Even in hospital it made some staff
uncomfortable to see me sitting up in bed, bald as a
badger, even though I was being barrier nursed. But I
just would refuse to toe the line.

Mark You said before you were told about damage to
your fertility. Now you're on oestrogen replacement.
So is there any chance you are fertile?

Christina No, absolutely zero.

Mark Does that worry you?

Christina It did, for a long time. And I think it was poorly
managed, too. Because of my age I needed to have
hormone replacement therapy almost straight away,
otherwise I would be osteoporotic in my forties. But it
didn't happen until quite a few years later, and it
meant me trying to find sympathetic endocrinologists.
Also I had the other side effects of low oestrogen, such
as a dry vagina. I guess that's what I mean by finding
sympathetic doctors. I found someone who was
fantastic and now I'm seeing someone else who's
equally as good. Very sympathetic, but professional
about it.

Mark Has that affected your sexuality? I don't just mean

the lack of oestrogen, but the whole business of having cancer at nineteen.

Christina Yes, yes it did. I think fertility often gets caught up in sexuality, and also in body image. It took me a long time to separate my sexuality from my fertility. But having done it, I've now got it worked out. But I don't think it's necessary to go through all the pain and suffering I went through. With professional intervention, it can be made easier.

And once I knew about IVF, I felt better. All I required was information. I knew there were donor oocytes. [Royal] North Shore [Hospital] has an IVF programme and they've used siblings. They've had a couple of successful pregnancies with oncology patients. I know the statistics and the success rate is only 11–12 per cent, but that's OK. It's not an issue at the moment, and I'm not sure I would subject my body to all that intervention again.

Mark Why? Are you worried that it might stir up the cancer or because you've been through enough?

Christina Because I've been through enough. I don't know that the need to have a child is paramount, although it would depend if my partner wanted to have one, I think. I'd definitely consider it. I've got lots of friends with children. I've got a brother and two sisters, and he's just got married, so I'm sure he'll have a child soon. I don't feel the need for me to have a child at the moment.

But I think sexuality and fertility is a huge issue, especially in my age group. It's one that's not dealt with at all, it's really swept under the carpet. And my oncologist was pretty callous in the way he told me, and that reflects his inability to deal with his own sexuality, I think.

Mark What did he say?

Christina I remember him saying 'Oh, by the way, you're going to be infertile'. This was after an hour long conversation about treatment, what I'd be having, side effects, and everything. It was very much a throwaway line at the end. The entourage left, and his registrar zoomed back in and said: 'Oh, by the way, don't get pregnant' and rushed out again. And that was it.

That's my perception. Maybe that's not exactly how it happened, but I was pretty devastated by that whole situation. When my treatment started it wasn't an issue, but when I went into remission it was a huge issue.

Mark Have you found any discrimination against you because you've had cancer? Friends, potential partners, work, anything? Have people turned away from you? Do they look at you differently?

Christina There was one girl at uni who found it difficult to cope. My friends at the time are still all my friends. It was really a learning experience for them as well.

Work? I think I was discriminated against once, but it's very hard to prove. I told this employer that I had had cancer, and in retrospect I don't think I would do that again. But you often have to have a medical, and I've had radiotherapy to my pelvis, back and front, so it's quite burnt and very obvious.

Partners. That's really tricky. Partners and friends, when do you tell them you've had cancer? It's letting them into a very personal part of your life, but the other side is that you have to deal with their reaction. 'Oh my God, cancer.' If they've had an experience of cancer, and a negative one because it's an elderly person who's died of their disease, then it's difficult. Once you get to know someone, that's when you tell them. Because I've got this huge chunk out of my life, and it's part of me.

I guess my experience of cancer was not all negative. It was difficult, and very taxing. Some really tough lessons to learn. But I think I've really changed my outlook.

For one thing, I was part of setting up CanYA.* And I've been much less materialistic—it's only recently that I've felt the urge to start acquiring possessions. Until this point they really haven't meant very much to me. It's the higher things in life—how you treat people, how you live your life. It all sounds a bit wanky, but I think having faced your own death, and my father's death as well, you realise that time is very precious. That, I think, accounts for my impatience. A lot of behaviour that you learn as a patient has to be unlearnt again, because once you're well again, it is not appropriate.

Mark   What sort of behaviour?

Christina   Being demanding, being very self-focused. You have to re-position yourself in a world where you're not the centre of the universe, you're just one person and while people around you seem to have very mundane lives, to them it's all very important. You can't just dismiss them as having no idea of what life is all about.

Mark   You tend to think that the rest of it is trivia?

Christina   Yes, I felt very detached from people. Part of the process of getting back into the land of the living was to really re-focus my outlook and stop looking so inward. But I guess I have experienced a lot of things that my peers haven't, and they won't experience until they are much older.

Mark   This book is mainly for parents. In what way can parents help their teenage kids?

Christina   I think it's very important people don't think there's a conspiracy and that information is not kept from either party. As I said before, I insisted on seeing my oncologist alone, as I felt our relationship was very personal, and it was between him and I, and my mother's reaction to that was that she was being shut

* CanYA is Cancer for Young Adults, a support for people with cancer aged between 20 and 35 years.

out. So he would see them separately. I was happy with that. He said he'd only discuss the same things with them as he discussed with me. We were all well informed—I think that's important.

It's very important for parents to allow their kids to be independent, even though the urge is to smother them and protect them, especially with a 20-year-old who's just starting out and trying new things and doing things that teenagers do.

A lot of the friction came from trying to maintain that balance. Dad did that better than Mum, although I guess I always had an easier relationship with him. He was very willing to accept me, and I guess he spoilt me a lot, too. But he'd done that because I was the first-born, and a daughter, and all that. Do you have any daughters?

Mark I have a first-born daughter. She's spoilt, but gorgeous.

Christina So he was more willing to let me go and to make my own mistakes, but to support me when I did make them. I moved out of home as soon as I could and went overseas about two months after I finished treatment. Even though I was really ill, they let me go. But Mum bought a ticket so she could come over and get me if I needed to be brought back, but I didn't.

I guess they let me make my own mistakes, and that was evident when they let me stop treatment. I had a friend with me and she told me the story quite recently.

I had just had my twenty-first birthday and she had come up for that from Melbourne. Apparently I walked out of my room and said to Mum that I wasn't having any more chemotherapy. Mum just picked up the phone and dialled the hospital and said 'Tina's not coming in today.' She said it was just like Mum saying that I had decided to stop eating butter and would eat margarine instead. There was no discussion and while

I'm sure she was quite distraught about the decision, she just accepted it. So they supported each other and were very much united in front of me. And they treated me like they had always treated me.

Mark Is there anything else you want to tell me about?

Christina Just that my rehabilitation process took a long time. Going into remission was just the start of that. The hard part was looking at my psychosocial needs—addressing my fertility and my sexuality and re-establishing myself in the world, going back to studying. They were all steps that I had to take.

The depression that followed me going into remission really needed some intervention. I was supposed to see my oncologist every three months and I refused to see him for a while, because I just couldn't bear to go to the hospital. But one day I decided I should see him and I rang him up and went along. That's how it went on. But I think people need to be supported at that stage. I'm not sure how that should happen, because you don't go to the hospital every week like you did for years. You can feel a bit lost.

And just treating the body isn't enough. You need to look after the soul or the spirit or whatever you call it as well. That took me a long time. It was really hard to get it back together. I think I'm there now but . . . that's about it.

Talking about the involvement of parents, I have a brother who is four years younger. He was sixteen at the time I was diagnosed. It was very difficult for him, because he had to grow up very quickly and look after my two younger sisters, who were twelve and eight.

Mum and Dad were away a lot and focused on me. I think he felt very left out and unloved. I'm sure they tried to compensate for that, and my two sisters don't really have any memory of being neglected at all, even though they were shunted from friends to relatives and all over, but Andrew did. He had lots of problems and when I was well again, we competed for attention and to reassert our positions in the family. We also had to re-establish our relationship, too. Family therapy, addressing those sorts of issues or at least acknowledging how difficult it is for siblings, would be really beneficial.

Also, I'm not sure how well informed he was. I'm sure he would have been, but I've never really asked him. That time I was up north and came back by air ambulance, I spent a night in Kempsey Hospital. It was thought at that stage that I was going to die, although I asked Mum recently if she was prepared for me to die and she said no. But my blood pressure was really low and my haemoglobin was 2.4* and it was all pretty catastrophic.

Andrew and my sisters and the poodle spent the night in the car in the hospital car park, and were taking Nicholas, the dog, for walks around the graveyard. Then they spent the next day at the hospital motel while I was being further stabilised until I could be shunted back to North Shore.

So there were lots of situations where he really had to be the man and deal with difficult situations. Then he cooked the duck on Christmas Day. I'm just not sure how much that was recognised and praised. I think parents should be very aware of other children, particularly the one closest in age to the patient.

Later, Christina expanded her thoughts on sexuality.

Christina I was diagnosed with cancer just before my twentieth birthday. I'd had several relationships with boys my own age but would have described myself as sexually naive and shy. My Catholic schooling and

* Normal haemoglobin is between 12 and 15 g/dL (grams per decilitre).

retiring personality certainly contributed to my sexual immaturity.

As I said before, the infertility caused by radiotherapy and chemotherapy was briefly and badly dealt with by my oncologist and his registrar. There were many other incidents during my treatment which added to my feeling of being uncomfortable with my body and not liking my body. For example, I had lower abdominal pain and went to casualty at the Royal North Shore Hospital. One of the examinations was an unsuccessful attempt by an orthopaedic registrar [who deals with bones] to perform a pelvic examination. Then while I was in hospital some staff members were offended by my baldness and would have preferred me to wear a scarf.

As well, the combination of chemotherapy and cancer meant I lost weight dramatically—photos taken at my twenty-first birthday remind me of a Belsen camp survivor.

On top of that, I went into menopause soon after I finished radiotherapy. I had hot flushes and so on. My oncologist prescribed hormone replacement therapy, but we didn't persist as the oestrogen made me feel nauseous. I didn't receive appropriate hormone replacement therapy until six years later.

For me, part of getting well involved disentangling my infertility from my sexuality. This meant getting accurate information about IVF and understanding some of the hormonal changes my body had been through. I finally found an understanding endocrinologist—the second endocrinologist I'd been referred to—who would talk frankly but kindly about my body. I felt comfortable enough to confide in her about my failed attempts at sexual intercourse. I saw a female gynaecologist who reassured me that my body was OK. So it was up to me to like, and finally love, my body.

It seemed much easier for me to deny that part of

my body than confront it. But a turning point was the official loss of my virginity just before my thirtieth birthday after three bottles of French champagne—I'm nothing if not stylish. The relief was immense. My body did work like everybody else's, even though as far as I'm concerned it still didn't and still doesn't look like everybody else's.

When do you tell a partner or potential lover that you have had cancer? That is very difficult. Relationships with doctors are certainly easier from that point of view, because they are much more likely to show fascination (do they intellectualise?) than fear and shock.

My image of my own body has improved dramatically over the years, as has my acceptance of the situation, past and present. I can now undress in a change room without being too self-conscious. I also had to confront my lop-sided pelvis when I started my sewing lessons. This rather simple process of making clothes has meant that I have learnt to accept my body. Although I'm not quite sure if I love it, yet.

Justin Cameron

Interview with Rhonda (mother), Alan (father) and Lauren (sister) Cameron at their home in Gatton, Queensland. This interview was carried out by Bruce Warren, a family friend and minister of the Uniting Church.

Justin was born on 10 January 1974. He was diagnosed with Ewing's sarcoma in April 1990. He had chemotherapy, surgery and radiotherapy. Biopsy confirmed that he had developed metastases in his lung in October. He died on 28 December 1990, aged 16.

Bruce   How do you think Justin really coped with the whole process?

Rhonda   On the whole he coped extremely well. Not only for him, but for everybody around him. Don't get me wrong—I'm not saying he didn't have all the fears and the anxiety that goes with it, but he remained positive and optimistic all the way through, no matter what he came up against. He could always find advantages over us.

Like his major operation, when he had to face such major surgery and the consequences of that surgery, he made out that he was going to be the advantaged one and we were going to be the disadvantaged ones after the surgery.

Within hours of him becoming paralysed, that was in the December, he was going to play wheelie basketball and swim for gold in the Disabled Olympics. He was a great swimmer, but he knew he was never going to be able to swim in the ordinary Olympics, but now he knew he was going to be able to swim for gold in the Disabled Olympics.

Bruce   Lauren, how did you perceive Justin coping with it?

Lauren   He helped me with it, because I knew he'd never look back. That helped me not give up and helped me keep going. When he became paralysed I was in Gatton and I can remember worrying about how he would be reacting and what he would be thinking. By the time I got through to Brisbane, I'd stopped worrying about that because he was not looking at the downside. He was looking at the good things about paralysis. That helped me a lot.

Bruce   Alan?

Alan   I guess Justin's reactions surprised me in a lot of ways. They were different to mine, obviously, as he was the one that was directly affected. I had a lot of times when I felt a certain way, or you'd come to Justin and you'd tell him something or you'd hear the doctors tell him something and your reactions would . . . you know, things would go through your mind. But already Justin would be coping with what he'd been told and already he was putting things into perspective in his life.

Because of his reaction and the way he dealt with these things, it made it a great deal easier for us. I think a lot of that was a conscious thing on his part, but it was also part of the way he was.

Rhonda That started right from day one, from the initial trip from Gatton to Brisbane after he'd had a shot of pethidine and we were told to put him in the car. We hoped it would bomb him out and he'd be there before the next lot was due. But all the way down, even when it was only a possibility of it being a tumour, even when we still thought it might be osteomyelitis [a bone infection], he was sitting in the car talking about the possibility of losing his hair from chemotherapy. And if it was cancer. Very calmly, very rationally, he'd already started to think and work out where he was going.

Alan And how he was going to handle it.

Rhonda Where I was just in a panic.

Bruce I'm going to ask you a hard one, because in our conversations previously we've talked about his positiveness and how determined he was. In your understanding, when do you think he understood he was dying?

Rhonda That is a hard one. We knew that if and when he developed secondaries, it was virtually maintenance treatment that he would receive. The primaries—fine, they could fight the primaries—but with the secondaries there was very little that could be done.

We had a two day wait for the results of his biopsy. It started to sink in that if those results came back positive, we would all have to rethink where we were going and how were doing it.

I was the one who had to break the news to Justin. That wasn't the most pleasant task. But still, even knowing that he had secondaries, he still, after we all had a cry and we all broke down and had a family hug, he immediately got back on with it.

From that point on, he actually said to me: 'Mum, I know what cancer is, but I still have today, and that's what I'm going to deal with—what is happening to me today. I will worry about tomorrow and what it brings when it comes.' So he didn't talk about his actual death, but he knew that he could die. He wasn't going to worry about the actual consequences of his illness until that time.

I believe that he said his goodbye to me the day before he died. Late that Thursday afternoon, he'd had a turn and he'd gone all vague, like he had the night before, when we had to rush him in on Boxing night, and he looked at me and he said: 'Mum, when I'm going, I am going.'

Because of everything that was happening at the time, I took it that his pain was increasing, and I asked him if he was in pain and did he need any more pain relief. He said no, but he loved me.

After that, he asked me to get the girls back to the room, Lauren and Vickki. They were on their way out of the hospital, but we had to send after them quickly to get them back. One of the nurses caught them just in time and they came rushing back. Justin settled after that and had gone into a sound sleep. Dr Beadle, the oncologist who was in charge of Justin's case, told us that he didn't know whether Justin would come out of that sleep and that optimistically we only had a few days left with him.

It was only a matter of five to ten minutes after the doctor left the room that Justin woke up. And the next six hours of that night were so precious, so normal, so almost a non-cancer situation. He was planning Lauren's birthday, which was in February, and he had lots of subtle, little requests that none of us picked up on at the time. I only realised later what he was doing.

He was just so happy and so normal. It wasn't as if we were in hospital. It was something special, very special.

Then he said he was tired and the girls went off—they were staying downstairs in the hospital that night—and he slept for an hour and the rest of that night, every fifteen minutes to half an hour, he looked at me and he asked me what time it was. He had never ever done that in the eight to nine months that we'd spent down there. It wasn't until the girls came back in that he brightened up, and it was only a matter of half an hour, 45 minutes later, before he just took his last breath.

I believe he knew, and I think he was ready, but that doctor coming in and giving us the news that he did, I really believe he hung on that little bit longer for us. I really believe that's what happened.

Bruce When you had to break the news to him about the secondaries, what were you feeling inside?

Rhonda It was just utter devastation. It was like I was dreaming, that it wasn't really happening. But he had to be told. He knew the results were coming through that afternoon. It couldn't be done as a family for Lauren's sake, because I had also had to break the news to him in June that his chemotherapy wasn't working because we were home and had to wait for the results here. I was the only one home that day . . . no, Lauren had arrived home from school but when Justin walked through the door, Lauren said: 'Mum, I've got to go,' and she just bolted until Justin had heard the news and then she came back into the room.

Bruce Lauren, what was happening for you that you felt you had to opt out?

Lauren I think it was just that I didn't know how Justin

was going to handle it. At that stage I still didn't want to face it. Seeing Mum tell Justin maybe would have made me face it, and that was something that I didn't want to do.

Bruce Alan, what about you? When that news was to be given, you were aware of it before Justin?

Alan No, Rhonda would have known before me. I would have been in Gatton.

Rhonda No, we were all in Gatton. You had to make the phone call and you rang me and you said: 'It's positive'. No, no, you didn't ring me and that's how I knew it was positive. Alan arrived home, and he didn't have to say anything because he wouldn't have been home if the biopsy wasn't positive.

Alan That's right, I was confusing it with the news about the chemotherapy. That time I had rung before I came home, but this time I thought I should come home first.

Bruce Rhonda, when you had to tell him about the secondaries, was there any sense in which you felt you failed him or that you were selling him out or somehow disappointing him as a mother, as a protector, as somebody who was trying to hold him together?

Rhonda I can remember he was lying on our bed when I told him, because I burst out crying first, which was probably a good thing because that made him cry and release some tension. Then Lauren came sneaking down the hall and I can remember him holding out his arms to include her in the hug. Then Alan was right behind her.

I didn't actually feel like I was selling him out, but I just felt so angry that it was him, and not me. I can remember telling him.

Going back to the chemo, that was the first time I told him that if there was any way possible that I could have traded places with him, to go through what he was going through, that I would have. And he told me that there was no way he would allow me to trade places with him even if I could have.

Maybe that's why I didn't feel that I had not protected him enough—we'd had these sort of talks all the way through. But I just felt so ... as though the inside was being ripped out from inside me. The utter helplessness ... that was when the helplessness really, really got to me.

Bruce Alan, what was running through your mind at this point? Were you feeling something similar to Rhonda or were you feeling something different?

Alan Probably similar to Rhonda in that you ask all the questions. Why? It had been explained to us that if the biopsy was positive and it was secondaries then it was, it was ... it was a matter of time, to put it bluntly. Rhonda used the word 'maintenance', and it means the same thing. They mean that's all they could do.

I thought it meant we still had some years. I thought it was possible we could keep it at bay for years. But even so, it was a fairly sudden jolt from what could have been perhaps a cure and a normal life thereafter to almost certainly a much shortened lifespan of one, two or three years. It turned out to be a couple of months.

But it was just ... you wondered what you could do. Why ... ? Up until then, we felt we had done all we could as far as medical treatment and hospitalisation and all that could be obtained was obtained. Now, what was left for us? I thought: 'What can we do now?'

Bruce But inside, what were you feeling at that moment when Rhonda had to break the news to Justin and you were all here, what were you feeling?

Alan Just ... it was almost as though we'd lost Justin already. We were virtually telling him that he was going to die. We felt that from this point on we were losing him. That's what I felt. This was the beginning of the end. However long it was, that was the start of it. You wondered what you could do, or how you could do anything.

Bruce You've talked about some of the hard parts. What were some of the parts that were made easy for you, and how did that happen? Lauren?

Lauren Justin's outlook made things a lot easier to deal with most of the time. His attitude changed my attitude. He taught each of us to live one day at a time. Yesterday is gone, so don't worry about it. Tomorrow's not here yet. Live for today and don't worry about anything else. He taught us to live each day to its fullest.

Bruce Rhonda, has it affected you the same way?

Rhonda Very much. The only way I survived was to focus on that day and not worry about what might happen. We didn't ask: 'What might happen next?' We faced what happened as it came, which was totally unnatural for me, because I was such a worrywart. The first thing I would normally like to know is what is likely to happen. But maybe because of the enormity of what we were facing, I ran away from that. I don't know.

Having heard Justin say what I was doing made it easier for me to do, because he voiced it, I heard it. We made pacts together. When I said goodnight to him after I told him about his secondaries, there was just the two of us in the room. We made a pact to fight harder. There wasn't much we could do at that point, but we made a point to fight harder.

I think what made it easier for us as a family was the total honesty. We didn't keep anything from Lauren at all.

Alan There were no pretends.

Rhonda Because of Justin's outlook on it, and not being frightened of the word 'cancer' or to say it, that meant we didn't have to be frightened of saying the wrong thing. We were more natural through those months than we ever had been in our lives. We didn't cover up anything.

Bruce How did that transfer over to other people—both immediate family and friends? How did you find it affected you in your relationships with them? Both prior to Justin's death, then afterwards. Alan?

Alan During Justin's illness, our relationships with friends and family and the community were quite good. There was support there from most avenues. We'd get the odd person who would avoid you for whatever reason—well, we knew the reason—but generally the support from the community and from our friends and our family was very good.

After Justin died, after the funeral, that changed. We are basically at a loss to know why.

Bruce Can you explain how that changed?

Alan I don't know whether it was a withdrawal of support, but people just weren't there. Where people would ring and call and so on, they just didn't come back after Justin died.

Bruce Did that concern you?

Alan Yes, yes.

Bruce How did you feel about that?

Alan I was hurt, but at the same time I tried to understand what they were going through. I guess Justin's death affected a lot of people who were supportive before he died, and it affected them in such a way that they didn't know how to talk to us or what to say. We were pretty new at the game ourselves, too.

Since then we've talked and heard and learnt from a lot of people and come to a lot of conclusions—these people really didn't need to do much at all except be there. They didn't have to say anything or do anything. But if you go back five years, we might have been the same. We'd never experienced anything like this. But once you've experienced it . . .

I perceive people who have lost a child since Justin

much differently to how I would have perceived them five years ago.

Bruce   Rhonda?

Rhonda   During Justin's illness it didn't affect me greatly as I was mostly in Brisbane with Justin anyway and surrounded by support from the hospital. And family and friends came to visit.

But I did notice when we were home occasionally that, especially if I was with Justin, that people who knew us well would avoid us. I knew that was because they didn't know what to say or how to face us.

It didn't worry me as much then as it did after we lost Justin. And it took me a long time to realise that some people hadn't been around. Close friends, who you would have expected to have called, hadn't. It was several weeks before it even dawned on me that there had been that gap. Then I felt very hurt, probably because it was a sudden realisation rather than a slower one.

I can identify very strongly with them not knowing how to deal with us, or wanting to give us space but at the same time, it doesn't stop the hurt.

Alan   You've lost your son, and you've lost your friends.

Bruce   Lauren, did you have any difficulties with schoolfriends or people you knew?

Lauren   During Justin's illness, when he had cancer, people wouldn't avoid me, but they wouldn't bring up the subject of Justin or cancer or anything.

After Justin died, I noticed a few people wouldn't come near me and if they did, it was just: 'Hello, goodbye.' But when I was around most of my friends, I didn't act abnormal or how they wanted me to act. I acted how I felt comfortable acting.

A few people were bit shocked by that, but most of them didn't worry. They wouldn't worry if I mentioned his name.

Alan   As Lauren said, she generally had good support

from her ten- or eleven- or twelve-year-old friends, which is something we missed out on from our thirty- or forty- or fifty-year-old friends.

Bruce Lauren, after Justin died, was there anything you felt you needed to do to make up that loss to Mum and Dad?

Lauren No, I didn't. All through, they didn't give Justin any more attention than me. Well, they did, but they still let me know that they loved me and cared for me. I didn't feel that I could make up for Justin.

Bruce Taking in everything that happened, can you see something that you have learned that you would not have discovered any other way?

Rhonda I've learnt to stand on my own two feet for the first time in my entire life. I guess the openness that we had from day one and continued to have right through ... Justin's positiveness, which led to our positiveness, gave me a feeling of self-worth. Most people expected me to fall in an absolute crumble right from the beginning. Few expected me to survive the months that we had to fight.

It's given me a feeling of being able to get up, get out and do something worthwhile. To really make something of time that I can give to help somehow, somewhere. This started back when Justin was having radiotherapy and I was sitting in the waiting room. I met a lady there during those weeks whose daughter had had cancer ten years earlier and she had survived.

The time I sat in that waiting room was when the clock started to tick over. I realised that I didn't have to be caught up with rushing around working. I could slow down, I could take time out, I could do something that I wanted to do that could help.

I talked about it even more when he became wheelchair bound. And Justin would say: 'Mum, you don't have to go to Brisbane to do things, we could raise money for cancer in Gatton.' Then with his paraplegia, we were

going to do all sorts of things. He talked along with me—
that has made the goals even stronger for me today. I
guess it's given me something to hang on to.

Bruce   Lauren?

Lauren   I've learnt to take one day at a time, like I said
before. Also, I never knew much about cancer. I used
to think that you lost your hair and died straight away.
But now I know that there's a lot more to it than that.
There's all the courage and the positive attitudes and
hope that's behind that. I've learnt a lot.

Bruce   Alan, what about you?

Alan   One thing, although I don't capitalise on it as much
as I should, is that I've learnt I've got a family who cares
about me and who cares about each other. I probably
don't make full use of that. Whether that's the trait of
a man, or the trait of a father, or the trait of just me,
I don't know. But it's certainly something that I've
learnt that I've got.

   That's probably the biggest thing I've learnt. All that
remains is to learn how to make the best possible use
of my family.

Rhonda   The one key that we had was honesty, total
honesty. Not just in Justin's diagnosis and his treatments, but our feelings. It was total honesty. It was
physical and emotional honesty.

Bruce   In terms of support systems, if you were to toss
around feeling and emotions and things that get at
you, where do you think you could go so you could get
this thing out on the table and work it through?

Rhonda   We were very lucky with the hospital that we had.
They were always one step ahead of what we needed,
and would offer or tell us what we needed to do about
getting whatever help, such as staying in Brisbane.

   They were giving us information before we even realised we needed it. We were never ever left floundering
during Justin's illness. We never came up against a situation where we would think: 'What are we going to

do about that?' The staff there gave us the information we needed to make whatever the next step was easier, before we even realised that we needed it. So we were very lucky in that regard.

Alan The hospital counsellors ... I don't think it's because it's a Uniting Church hospital, but a nurse counsellor was made available to Justin and Rhonda, and particularly since Justin's death we'd see this guy once a month as a family group.

It's two or three or even four months since we've seen him, but that was one place that we know it's only a matter of a phone call and we can lob in Brisbane and we've got this guy who will sit with us for any length of time. I guess he knows what we want to talk about before we do, before we even speak.

Bruce Would you say it's crucial to have that sort of support after the event?

Rhonda Definitely. I got to know him before Jus died by joining in the staff relaxation sessions they have. As time went on, Justin joined in when he was mobile, then when he was confined to bed this guy would come down and put Justin through a relaxation session on his own, in bed. We weren't ... I guess we were getting some sort of counselling without really knowing it, but we weren't having counselling sessions as such. We were having relaxation periods which were absolutely wonderful.

Then we've had lots of help from the Compassionate Friends and the local grief group here afterwards. Without that help, of being able to talk to people who knew what you meant, knew where you were coming from, it wouldn't have been so easy ... oh, I don't mean easy. It's not easy.

Alan You wonder what might have happened.

Rhonda Yes, you felt low enough as it was, but to be able to talk to somebody who really knew how you felt without even having to finish the sentence, just brought so much comfort that we were normal, that there were other people who felt the same. Definitely essential.

Christine Griffin

Interview with Jan Griffin in her Brisbane home, about her daughter Chrissy. Chrissy was born on 7 April 1965 and died on 16 May 1981, at the age of 16. Other family members: husband Frank and daughters Kathryn, Tricia, Claire, Lisa and Linda.

Jan She had a sore shoulder, but she was in the Girl Guides and they have a march each Anzac Day to the local park. Because she was one of the leaders, she carried the flag. We thought she'd strained her shoulder.

It went on for about a week and it seemed as though it wasn't getting any better, so we took her to the doctor. He originally still thought it was some kind of strain from carrying the flag. That would have made it about a month, I guess.

Then one day she was trying to put her blouse on, and it was really hurting. I thought it wasn't right— she should have been getting better. So I got a referral to an orthopaedic surgeon and by chance we were able to see him the next day. He had a cancellation. He X-rayed her and knew straight away. He put her straight into hospital. She had an operation [a biopsy] that night, and that's when we found out what it was.

It was completely out of the blue. She was a normal fourteen-year-old girl who played netball and swam and did lots of sport. She was good at school. We had no idea what hit us.

It was really worse, because exactly twelve months before I had been diagnosed with lymphoma, and that's why I was very jumpy about this lump. I said to the doctors at the time that I was a bit paranoid about lumps.

Mark She had a lump as well as the pain?

Jan It really wasn't noticeable until pretty close to when it was diagnosed. It was more that it was sore. I think they found it pretty quickly, really.

But when that lump turned out to be what it did, we were absolutely distraught, because at the time when I was diagnosed, I'd had a diagnostic laparotomy and the surgeons told my husband 'I'm sorry, there's nothing further I can do for her', so we'd gone through all this exactly twelve months before. But I went on chemo and it worked like magic. So I was frantic. I couldn't believe lightning could strike twice.

Mark Were you still having chemo at the time?

Jan No, I was better. But it was almost twelve months to the day. The night of Chrissy's operation was the middle of June—the longest night of the year. And it was the longest night, because I cried all night.

They decided when she had that operation that it wasn't like having it in the leg, where she could have her leg off. They felt there wasn't any surgery they could do.

She came home and Dr Martin arranged for me to see Peter Smith, he's a professor now, but he was in charge of the oncology ward at Royal Children's Hospital in Brisbane, and he's absolutely marvellous.

When she was over the surgery—we had to do sterile dressings on her shoulder, as it took months and months for her to heal—we went to QRI [Queensland Radiation Institute] for her to start having radiation, and she started her chemo at about that time.

She had six weeks of radiation. The first six months of the chemo were worst. I think she had only adriamycin for the first six months, and it was the worst. It made her the sickest. It made her lose her hair, too, which is probably the worst thing for a girl at that age. But then, she was good about it. She was good about everything, really. She was probably better than we were. She was amazing. She was so brave.

People seem to say that. I don't know whether children are given extra strength to cope, but I've seen other people that have lost their children and they've all said the same thing—about how brave they are.

I guess being a teenager was harder. It was before the days of CanTeen and that sort of thing. She always felt out of place. QRI was full of old men in their checked dressing gowns with lung cancer. She loved the doctor and the staff at the clinic. And there was a rocking horse at the clinic, and soft toys, but she was too old. It's good that since then, they've got the teenagers together. It makes it easier for them. Apart from the odd time, she really didn't meet any people her own age with cancer.

The chemo was pretty grim. She used to get dreadfully sick for a day or two after she'd had it. But she did fairly well with it. About twelve months later she ran in the cross-country at school.

Everyone at the clinic was as distraught as we were when she got the recurrence, because they all thought she'd done so well.

Mark At that stage you thought she'd been cured?

Jan Well, we hoped. We knew she had to have two years' treatment … I don't know. My husband always thought she'd get better, but I wanted to wait until the treatment was over before I thought that.

I've got one daughter who's a nursing sister and another who's a radiotherapist, so obviously we knew a fair bit about it. And I read all the books I could find. They said that with Ewing's she only had about a 5 per cent chance—I don't know if the percentages have improved since then. So I didn't dare hope. I wasn't pessimistic, but I wanted to see how she was going after the two years.

But she started getting pains in her back. For a long time they didn't find it. She had bone marrow things and all sorts of tests done, and each of them would come back negative. We kept hoping that it hadn't come back. That went on for a month or so, then she got worse and they had to admit her to hospital.

When she was admitted she gradually got worse. They phoned me one morning and said one of her vertebrae had collapsed and she was getting pins and needles. She went straight to surgery then.

They did this operation where they went in through her chest and they found that it had recurred. They did some kind of a bone graft on her spine. She was able to walk until the day she died. I didn't realise at the time what a marvellous operation that was. We were all so upset to know for sure that it definitely was a recurrence. We suspected it—we virtually knew it had to be. But the tests kept coming back negative and giving us fresh hope.

From then on, she had metastases in her leg. Probably the worst of all was that she had to have her CAT scan and it was, well it was either in her brain or in her head. I was frantic about that because we'd had some friends whose son had died from a brain tumour and we knew what that was like. I couldn't bear to think of Chrissy like that. She'd had such great spirit through it all, she tried so hard. If she could drag herself out of bed and go to school, she would. She went to school right up to between six weeks and a month before she died. That was what was so good about the operation— she was able to walk and do all those things.

My sister came over at Christmas from New Zealand, and Chrissy was talking about her sixteenth birthday party. I'd just heard about it going to her brain or head or whatever, and when my sister went back she said she'd live to that party. I didn't think she would, I thought she only had a few weeks. They'd said then that it was a matter of weeks, rather than months.

But she did. She made it to her sixteenth birthday, had a party with all her friends, then ... I think that's what she was waiting for. People can do that, you know.

I can't remember when they stopped treatment. I nursed her at home until the Saturday—she was in hospital for the last five days because one of the best things they did for me was to teach me to give pethidine injections. She wasn't waiting for the Blue nurses to come. Dr Smith said there was no upper limit for it—she was to be kept painfree. I was a lab technician before I was married but I wasn't a nurse—I'd never given an injection in my life. They taught me to give one in an orange first. Then my husband was there, he went very pale, but he was my first victim. I gave him one. I got to be really good at it because I gave so many of them. I think Chrissy preferred me to give it.

As well as me there was Tricia, who's a nursing sister, and there's a friend across the road who's a nursing sister. She used to give them until they taught me. In that respect we were very lucky because having a big family like we have, there was always someone around. It wasn't just the close family—there was my husband's sisters and brothers-in-law and my sisters and everybody rallied around a fair bit to help—and friends and neighbours. Lisa and Linda were only little girls then and people used to pick them up from school for me if I was at the hospital. Everybody helped me a lot. I was a lot luckier than somebody who had to come down from the country away from family and friends.

Chrissy's friends were very good, too, throughout the two years. Her schoolfriends and other friends were great. They were always ringing her up and visiting her—they were all very loyal.

When you look back on it you wonder how you ever

coped. We had a wedding in the middle of it—our eldest daughter was married and that was the week I'd heard about it going to the head. I don't know how I managed to put on a wedding, but we did.

Chrissy had just had the big spinal operation and she was in a cast and she was flat on her back. There was this lovely old sister—I shouldn't call her old, she might have been younger than me—who was in charge of Turner Ward; Sister Guthrie. She'd been there for donkey's ages. Kathy and her husband and all the bridesmaids were going up to the hospital to visit. But Sister Guthrie got the idea this wasn't good enough. Chrissy had to go to the wedding.

She arranged for a special chair that they take the paraplegics out in to come over from Prince Alfred Hospital, because Chrissy was in the Children's. The ambulance couldn't take her because they can't just take people to a social occasion. My son-in-law had a Kombi, but he was the groom. So we had to arrange things.

My brother-in-law drove the Kombi. He and his son carried Chrissy in the chair into the Kombi. My sister-in-law went up and dressed her for the wedding, and my friend across the road went in case she needed an injection on the way to the wedding. She looked after her through the wedding. So she was able to come to the wedding—it was just wonderful for her to be there. I didn't think she'd be able to come. That was really good. She had a few glasses of champagne at the wedding—she reckoned she was the only one who ever went back to the Children's Hospital a bit tipsy.

And poor Tricia was sitting for her nursing finals on the Monday Chrissy went into hospital, just before she died, so between all of that ...

The reason she went into hospital then was that on Mother's Day, which was the Sunday night, she had this ... I don't know what you'd call it, but she couldn't breathe. By this time it had gone to her lungs. She couldn't breathe and she was sort of choking. Tricia was here—she did something that got us through that, but I thought that was really beyond me. I couldn't cope. I'd managed all the nursing, but I was worried for her sake.

Also, she was getting more pain. So when she went into hospital, they put a drip in with morphia, which meant she didn't have to have injections all the time. She went to hospital on the Monday morning and she died on the Saturday morning. I'd stayed the night at the hospital the night before and my husband came up in the morning and I'd gone home to have a shower and get changed. He was with her. He said she just slipped away. By that stage she was sleeping a lot.

We were all sitting around the bed one day and we were all crying, because she was asleep. She woke up and she said: 'You're a weepy wailing lot.' So we all cheered up a bit. She had this fighting spirit. I think she knew she was going to die, but she didn't seem to want to talk about it. You always read in all the books that you should talk about it, but I don't think she wanted to. She might have talked to other people . . .

Mark   Did she talk to her friends about it?

Jan   I don't think so. She went out for dinner one night with Claire and the boyfriend she had then. She said to him: 'Are you coming to my funeral?' That put a bit of a dampener on the evening.

I'm sure she talked to the people in the hospital, because a couple of the doctors who had been registrars and had moved on to different areas still used to come and see her quite a bit. I think she talked to them rather than talk to us about it. The only thing she ever said in front of me was that she didn't want people to forget her. I don't think there's much chance of that. I think more people remember her because she was sick, or she made more friends, or impressed more people, than if nothing had ever happened to her.

But I don't think she said anything to the family apart from that. Claire didn't even tell me about her asking Peter if he was going to come to her funeral until after she'd died. She said she wanted a big funeral, too, and she got that wish. The church was packed.

She was so ill at the end that there's worse things than dying. She was so ill. She had a spare bed in her room and I moved in there in case she needed me during the night. It was so hard for her to breathe. You really don't want them to go on living like that.

Mark It was a relief in the end?

Jan I felt so. It was great that she just slipped away. One of my fears was that ... one of my husband's aunties was a nun and she died of lung cancer. Don't ask me why she got lung cancer—I'm sure she never smoked in her life. We were all around the bed when she died, and that was awful. I thought maybe that was what was going to happen because it had metastasised to her lungs. But she didn't. Frank said she was sleeping and she was breathing and then he said to the nurse: 'She's stopped breathing.' She just slipped away.

And Kathryn, my eldest daughter, said: 'She's got her long blonde hair back, now.' I guess that's the way we think about her now.

I did have her two school photos from the year after that when she had really short hair. She did have a wig. I don't know whether wigs have improved, but they looked like wigs and she hated wearing that. She wore a wig to school and when she was going out, and when she was home she just took it off. She didn't like caps and scarves. You always knew if you were a really good friend or not, because she didn't bother to put it on if she liked you.

And she had such a pretty face that it didn't matter.

She looked really cute when her hair first came back. In fact, somebody stopped her in the bus and asked her where she got her hair cut, because she wanted to get a haircut like that. But as I say, when she had the steroids it changed her appearance.

Mark   What was the thing she was most scared of?

Jan   Towards the end she hated going for the chemo because she knew she was going to get sick. I couldn't even talk about it because if I'd say we were going on Monday to start again, well, she didn't want to hear that. She used to get sick before she even got there. And she hated losing her hair.

But as far as being really scared, she never let on if she was. Obviously she must have been scared of dying, everybody must be scared of dying, but she never said much.

I think she hoped pretty much until the last lot of chemo. Then she said: 'It doesn't seem to be doing much good' or: 'It'd better hurry up' or something like that.

Mark   Did she just accept it as her lot?

Jan   She tried to pretend she was like everyone else. She didn't want to be sick or different in any way.

Mark   Did she want you to treat her like you were treating everybody else?

Jan   Yes, she didn't want anybody to fuss over her or to talk about it. When she got really sick, you think of things like: 'Should we take her to Lourdes?' Or there are people who come in and lay their hands on. We're Catholic, but there are people like that.

But I think she'd have hated that. She didn't want to be taken to Lourdes and treated like an invalid, or being sick. She just wanted to be like everybody else.

She insisted I went up and bought all her schoolbooks for grade 11, and we didn't even know she'd get back to school that year. She did get back for nearly five months. That was one of the hardest things I had to do—go up to the school and buy her books when I knew jolly well that she wasn't going to be using them.

She got a very good Junior Certificate even though she missed a lot of school through being ill. She was really determined she should get it. I had to get in touch with the headmistress and make sure she'd done all the exams and assessments that she needed to do so she could get her Junior Certificate.

Mark There must have been an enormous strain on your family. Do you think the other girls missed out in some ways?

Jan We did the best we could. The little girls certainly didn't know she was going to die. I tried to be everything to everyone, I guess. I tried to make sure nobody missed out.

Lisa had to get her appendix out during the time Chrissy was quite ill. Lisa had to go to hospital with appendicitis. I think she thought that was marvellous because she was getting all the attention and the toys and things like that which, well, Chrissy got spoilt. There's no two ways about it.

So maybe they felt . . . But there's so many of us. Kathryn was twenty-one and Tricia was eighteen. They were old enough, if I wasn't here, to look after the younger ones. It was probably very hard on Claire, working at Queensland Radiation Institute and knowing full well what was going on. I'm sure it was hard on all of us. You'd have to ask them if they felt they missed out. I think we all did the best we could, particularly for Chrissy. She was the one who needed us. We didn't need that much, really.

I found with Linda, after Chrissy died, that she worried. She was eight. She's got long blonde hair and she looks very much like Christine. I guess we all lose hair in our comb, but she seemed to lose a lot of hair. She used to worry about her hair falling out, and she used to get pains in the stomach.

I realised what she was thinking. She thought that because her hair was falling out, she had cancer. I was pleased that I realised that was what she was thinking, and I could explain to her what happened with hair falling out and so on. Because it would have been worse if she had kept bottling it up.

We're a pretty close family. I think we helped each other through and we helped each other afterwards. You never get over it. There's always a big hole in the family. But we're not really a sad family.

I've heard of some situations where there's been nervous breakdowns afterwards and families have split up after a tragedy. But I don't think we've had anything like that here.

Mark Did you make a special effort to maintain your relationship with your husband?

Jan I did the best I could. He was very busy at work. I think he would have liked to have done more as far as nursing Chrissy goes, but he was always pretty busy at work. I don't think there were ever any real problems. We'd been married 22 years. We had a very stable marriage that could weather the storms. Everybody missed out a bit because she came first, but I wouldn't like to think they missed out too much. And they'd be upset to think they should have been getting extra attention. They were quite happy to help out as best they could.

Mark How did your friends and relatives react?

Jan I can only think of one fairly good friend who didn't do much. Most of my friends were marvellous. They did what they could to help out. Yvonne was probably my greatest help throughout, as far as a friend is concerned. She was always thinking up little surprises for Chrissy and buying her little things, and looking after her if I had to go out. Because she was a nursing sister we were quite confident to leave her with Yvonne, although I never left her much. Between the family there was usually somebody here, because all the girls were here for the most of it. Kathy got married six months before Chrissy died, but there's a lot of us.

As far as Chrissy's friends were concerned, there was only one who Chrissy used to call her fair weather friend. She never used to come and see her much when she was sick and had no hair, but when her hair grew back and she looked really cute and all the boys loved her, this other girl used to ring up all the time and want to go out places with her.

But the rest of her friends were pretty loyal to her. She had one particular friend, Donna, who lived at the back. They'd grown up together from when they were babies. She was always there for her to talk to. They were very close.

Mark Is there anything else you want to talk about?

Jan Well, I wish they could get something that would make chemotherapy easier. I've had chemotherapy and I did get sick, but not like she was. Poor Chrissy, she said: 'Mum, I never realised how sick you were. I wish I'd known, then I would have done more for you.'

I feel maybe the wrong one got better. But I guess not. I would have preferred it was me, because I could cope when I was sick. I didn't worry much about myself. I guess people worried about me, but I didn't worry about myself. I always thought I was going to get better.

But it's a lot harder when it's your child. It's very difficult for parents. You hate to see your kids sick.

[Lisa arrived]

Mark How old were you at the time?

Lisa I was eleven when Chrissy died. I don't know how old I was when she first got sick.

Mark Did you have much idea of what was going on?

Lisa Not really. I knew she was sick, but I didn't even know what she had until I got older. I don't remember very much about it.

Mark   Was it a big event in your life?

Lisa   It was a really big thing. We quite often used to go to the hospital with Mum and all that. It was a really big thing, but ...

Mark   Did you feel there was much change in the way the family operated while she was sick?

Lisa   Obviously, we didn't see Mum as much as before she got sick, because Mum was spending a lot of time with Chrissy. And I stopped sharing a room with Chrissy when she got really sick, so that was a change.

It was weird for a while after she died, because we weren't used to not having her around.

Mark   How old are you now?

Lisa   Twenty-two.

Mark   Do you think the whole thing made you any different to your friends?

Lisa   It's funny. It made me feel a bit more sure that God existed. I was a Catholic, and we were supposed to think that there was a heaven and a God ... sorry, I don't usually cry ... but after Chrissy died I knew I was supposed to think that there was an afterlife and a God. And that when you died you would be with God and it would all be great, but I never really thought it was true. I thought you died, and you just weren't there any more. But after Chrissy died I couldn't stand to think that she didn't go anywhere, so it really changed the way I thought about God and dying.

Ever since she died, I've prayed to Chrissy. We all do it. So that was one big impression it made on me. It changed the way I think about my religion.

Mark   So making the decision that heaven had better exist helped?

Lisa   Yes, for sure. It was comforting.

Jan   When we were out at the cemetery it was quite still, and then this wind whipped up. My sister-in-law said it was Chrissy having a look to see who was there, and making sure we all knew she was up there watching it.

Mark Does going to the cemetery help?

Jan No.

Lisa No.

Mark You don't feel like she's there?

Jan No, she's in heaven. I felt duty-bound to go on her birthday and anniversaries and Christmas, and we take flowers, but it upsets me. I prefer to keep flowers by her picture and look at her the way she was, and to believe that she's in heaven. I'd rather think she's in heaven than out at the cemetery.

Lisa The cemetery is always funny because there's this 96-year-old woman on one side and a two week old baby on the other. I always think that's really sad.

Jan I feel very close to Chrissy beside the sea, because she always liked surfing and we always spent our holidays beside the sea. We spent a lot of time by the sea. It was always a place where she was happy.

   [Tricia arrived]

Mark How old were you at the time Chrissy was diagnosed.

Tricia I was four years older than Christine, so I must have been eighteen. I was in my first year of nursing when Christine was diagnosed? She was sick for two years and she died the Saturday before, no after, my nursing finals.

Mark Did you think at the time you had particular problems because you were nursing?

Tricia Oh yes, definitely. Working in a paediatric ward was particularly difficult. In fact all oncology patients were difficult, because I could relate it to the family situation.

Mark Was more expected of you because you were a nurse?

Tricia A lot was expected of me. When she was first diagnosed, she had a biopsy on her shoulder. The wound broke down, and she also had radiation burns. She needed daily or twice daily dressings, and the wound needed packing. I was able to do dressings by that stage, and when she became terminally ill Mum and I took turns night about, to give her intramuscular analgesia. She was having about 200 mg of pethidine two hourly towards the end. I think Mum and I shared the nursing of Christine towards the end. The other girls were a bit ... Well, Claire was doing radiography but I think she was a bit scared to spend the night with Chrissy when she was really sick.

Mark Did you find it hard to separate your roles as sister and nurse and resident medical expert?

Tricia Definitely, yes. When Chrissy was first diagnosed, I knew a lot more than Mum ever knew because I went straight to work and looked it up. I saw the mortality rate and saw it was fairly serious.

There were a few occasions where I knew they were secondaries before the others. When she had the back pain we were told it might be osteomyelitis [a bone infection]. But why would she be getting osteomyelitis when she had Ewing's sarcoma? That was the first sign of metastases—pain in her back. So I guess that with my access to medical books, I knew a bit more. And I suppose it was difficult to separate out the roles.

I remember one occasion, it was a family party for Julie's birthday and Christine was having trouble breathing, and everybody said immediately: 'Tricia, what do we do?' I thought: 'Oh my God, what do I do?'

We sat her up and eventually she caught her breath, but it was terrible. I just couldn't think of what to do in a hurry. It's very difficult to be a nurse to your sister. It's very easy to separate your emotions from a patient because you don't know them and you've had nothing to do with them, but even sponging Christine, I'd be more anxious to please and worried that I was doing it right. And I never wanted to hurt her while doing the dressings, where with a patient you're not so emotionally involved and you don't get so upset if it's not done right. It was a very hard time all round.

Mark   How has Chrissy's experience changed your life?

Tricia   It's definitely changed my life, but I can't say specifically in what way. I'm probably more empathetic to people who have lost a family member, and there's obviously a big void in your life when you're one of six girls and there's only five. We always think of her, all the time.

But it's more losing Chrissy that has affected my life, rather than anything else from around that time. It affects you in every way. You miss her, you wish it had never happened, in your work it affects the way you deal with patients. I'm doing midwifery, and probably one of the reasons I'm doing it is that not many people die. I couldn't stand to be in the situation where people die all the time. I found that very depressing when I was there.

I probably get too involved with some of the babies that die. But at least it's a happy feelgood area most of the time. But I couldn't stand working in an oncology ward. I don't know how people do it.

It must have been hard for Claire doing radiotherapy. She would have been faced with people every day that had cancer. In fact, when she was interviewed, Christine had had Ewing's and I think they were a bit reluctant to take her on because she'd be dealing with so many oncology patients. It must be terribly hard for her, but maybe she's the sort of person ... I just couldn't do it.

Karen Knight

Interview with Janet, Frank and son Bruce Knight in their Brisbane home about their daughter Karen. Karen was born on 23 August 1971 and died on 13 October 1991. She was aged 20.

Frank   The first thing was the pain in her back. We put it down to training, because she was a hurdler and she was doing the long hurdles. The university physio treated her for muscle strain for about two months.

Janet   She'd just started some weights, too, so she was always sore. Being sore from time to time was just part of training.

Frank   I was actually massaging her back, and I didn't find any lumps at all.

Janet   She didn't complain of one sore spot. Just soreness. Then she was asked to coach at a school in an outback town one weekend, and she went out there with a couple of other young ones. She got some real pain in her back and she had to go to the hospital. That wasn't like her, because she was pretty tough.

The next week she came home from training on the Monday night and said 'Oh, there's a burning in my back. A real burning.' I was working at the time, and she was too—we used to work in the same building. So we took a day off work and we went to the local doctor. He sent us for X-rays at the Prince Charles Hospital. He must have suspected something because he didn't just send us to an ordinary X-ray place.

We brought them back and he saw us that night. They didn't show anything at all—they were clear. But he knew there was something wrong, and he got her in for a scan next day. That was pretty unusual. You usually have to wait a week or so. The scan showed some sort of a mass.

Mark   Apart from her sore back, was she healthy at the time?

Janet   Yes, yes.

Frank   She was in very good condition.

Janet   She was probably looking at her best. She was really strong. She had grown again. She was fairly tall, about 5'11' [1.80 cm], and through all her growth spurts she would normally look pretty thin, before she'd fill out again. But this time she had looked really strong. She was training for the 400 m hurdles, and that's a hard event to do.

She didn't have any other symptoms at all. But it all accelerated from just a soreness to just one spot.

Anyway, the scan showed there was something there, so she was admitted to hospital next day and they did a needle biopsy of it. We had to wait two or three days to find out that it was malignant, and they said they had to take it out. It was about the size of a softball.

It was about a week from the time she went to the doctor and had the X-ray to the time she had the operation. They established in the operation that it was all over the eleventh rib, and it had attached itself to the tenth and the twelfth, too. So they had to take three ribs.

Because that left such a huge hole there, they had to support her lung by what they described as a stretchy piece of gauze. Also, they had to put a piece of something similar over her kidney, because it was exposed.

She spent five days in intensive care, then another week in the postoperative ward. Then we were told what it was. We had to wait almost a week and a half, almost two weeks, before we knew what it was and whether there was going to be any treatment. The surgeon assured us that the area was clear and he was quite pleased with the way the operation went.

But when she recovered sufficiently, they wanted to re-scan her whole body. They scanned her lungs three times, because they weren't sure. They told us the scan mightn't have been a good job, and they couldn't establish whether these little marks they saw were just movement at the time of the scan or what. But they finally told us that they were dozens of small tumours inside both lungs.

That was bad. They told us she had to have eighteen

months of chemotherapy and hopefully that would be able to knock over the tumours.

It was devastating for her and for us, but we sort of accepted that. We thought 'Oh well, that's OK.' We knew it would change her life completely, and she would have to give up athletics, which was devastating for her. That was absolutely terrible for her. The other thing that was devastating for her was that she was going to lose her hair. She had long blonde hair.

But, we seemed to take it as it came. She got over the operation, and she was up walking . . .

Mark At that time you had been told what was going on. What were your thoughts in the time between the scan and when you found out?

Janet Well, we weren't all that worried because immediately after the operation, the surgeon came out and told us that he was pleased with the job and that the area was clear. He had taken a big area, and the outer rim had been tested and it was clear. Not being medical people, it didn't occur to us that it might be in the bloodstream somewhere else. We thought 'Well, that was cancer, and she's been cleared of cancer.' We didn't think any further than that.

Frank We were even told that Ewing's was one of the curable cancers. That's what we were told by the hospital.

Janet And one of the doctors we knew was being positive. They were all being positive. They were saying it was curable.

Frank Then later we found out how aggressive it can be, and how hardly anyone who has had secondaries can survive it. The problem with that cancer is getting it before the secondaries get out. It's the sort of cancer you never know anything about until it's too late, and we were told she'd had it some time. They explained at the hospital how it grew and the time it took to get to the stage where they could pick it up on scans.

Janet So she'd had it for some time. But how on earth would you know? She was healthy as anything—really healthy.

Frank You don't just go and have a scan for no reason, do you? It's not the sort of thing you walk in off the street and have. That's the part that really surprised us. I was shocked. Shocked. And you end up blaming yourself for not picking it up earlier.

I'd been pretty involved with sport for a while. I've been to many many lectures on sporting injuries, and I pick up quite a few sporting injuries, but I didn't pick this up. The physio didn't pick it up, either, and he'd been working with her for a couple of months.

Janet But she'd only been occasionally. In that two months she'd only been four or five times, and she continued training. At that stage it didn't jar her to run or to walk or anything like that, so it really escalated quickly. In that week before the operation it got bad all of a sudden.

So with the news that she had to have eighteen months of chemotherapy, the bottom just dropped out of everything. We wondered 'what now for the future?'

She was working, and we knew she had to give up work. She was working in an office—it was a typing service but it was a stationery office as well. Because of her commitments with the sport, she was just a bit different from other girls of that age.

Frank It took up a lot of her time.

Janet Yes, it did. And she had to work at something or study something that gave her time for athletics. Athletics was first to her. But we knew and she knew that it was only a sort of temporary thing, because there's no such thing as a full-time athlete in Australia. You've got to have a job. But she knew that. Being young as she was, she wanted to put her best foot forward and put everything into it for a few years.

We still don't know what she would have done. She wanted to be a hairdresser, but ... her whole life was athletics.

Mark So the treatment was mapped out for you—eighteen months.

Janet Yes. She had the drugs every three weeks. We were told about the drugs and the side effects, and that she might be hospitalised in between treatments because her blood count would go down to almost nothing and she might contract an infection.

That's exactly what happened after the first treatment. Because it was an aggressive cancer, and because they were trying to knock over the tumours in her lungs, they were going to administer the strongest doses they possibly could according to her weight and age.

They did that all right. It only took one lot of chemotherapy and she lost all her hair. She was hospitalised between the first and second lots of treatment with an infection and a high temperature.

Mark How did she handle losing her hair?

Janet When she was told she would lose her hair she accepted it, because we were talking about a wig. When her hair did start to fall out, she was in hospital because of that infection. That was probably for the best, because the staff there were so good. They consoled her a bit. But she just accepted it.

Mark Did she wear a wig or a scarf or go bald?

Janet She wore a wig. She wore a cap, too, at home. But she wore a wig that looked almost identical to her hair.

Frank It didn't stop her social life. She'd come out of hospital and be out socialising next day.

Janet She loved the night life. She was a real wild dancer. She lived dangerously. She would always be conscious of her blood count, but there were a few occasions where she took the risk and it would work out OK. It didn't stop her going on living.

Frank She still trained occasionally.

Janet Yes, not to the same extent, but she did go out to meetings and training with the squad. It didn't stop her doing much at all. We look back now and we think that was good.

Mark During that eighteen months, how did she react to the three-weekly cycle?

Janet Well, it was only eleven months from the time she was diagnosed to the time she died, and it was only the first eight months that she had any quality of life.

    She didn't like to go back, but she knew it was only one or two nights away and she'd be back, then she'd have a couple of sick days after that then she'd be right.

    She was just accepting. She knew she'd have to do it and then it would be over and done with. Because she didn't have any commitments. Training was no longer ... you know ... and she didn't go to work, so she didn't have any real commitments. She was fairly accepting of it, and she never complained. You know how people will often say that patients never complained, but they really did, well, she honestly never complained. She didn't once say 'Why me?' Not once. Did she Frank?

Frank No. The treatment was working for about six months. It was clearing her lungs. But then they found the treatment wasn't going to continue to work, so they tried something else.

Janet They changed the drugs, because they found she had pain in her spine. It had come back in her spine.

Mark It sounded like things got a lot better. Did you think then that she was going to be OK?

Frank Yes. Right to the end, I never really believed it was going to kill her.

Janet At the beginning, it didn't occur to me and I don't think it occurred to anyone—it certainly didn't occur to Karen—that she might die.

Frank   When the doctors called us in and told us that it had gone to the spine and they were going to change the drugs, even then I didn't believe ... I didn't ... even then I was hopeful. Even at that stage, right up until a month before.

Janet   Well I wasn't, nor was Karen. We just ... accepted the inevitable. That's not to say we gave up, but she needed some support. I just felt it was no good saying everything was going to be all right. She was too old for that. She was nineteen. She wanted to know everything and she was told everything. That's the way she wanted it.

Mark   Who did the doctors deal with—Karen or you?

Janet   I was there all the time. I didn't stay the night, because it wasn't the sort of hospital where you did that.

Frank   It was basically her looking after herself and you helping, wasn't it?

Janet   Yes. And there was never any of this being called outside the room and whispering behind her back, was there? She was told everything, and she asked plenty of questions.

The doctors hadn't told us too much. Obviously they hadn't. When I look back now I'm pleased they didn't, because we would have been in a panic.

I don't know why we did it when she had just gone so many months and things seemed to be improving— I guess we just wanted to find out more about this— but even before she started to get bad, we went in to the Queensland Cancer Fund's library. You can't take anything out of that library, so we were there for half a day and we looked through a lot of things.

Mark   You said you were glad you weren't told everything at the start. Why?

Janet   Ignorance is bliss sometimes.

Mark   Do you think the treatment and everything Karen went through was worth it?

Janet   Yes, because I think it prolonged her life by three or four months. Don't you think so?

Frank   Yes, because there were fewer tumours there when she had a scan at six months than originally.

Janet   I'd say it prolonged her life by four months or so.

Mark   Do you think she thought it was worth it?

Janet   Yes. She was a real livewire. Karen went through a lot with treatment. She was sick, and it wasn't very good, but it was only a few days out of three weeks and the rest of the time she was pretty good.

Mark   Talking to different families, they all have their own way of dealing with cancer. Did you concentrate on Karen because she was sick, or did you try to make sure the other kids were looked after? How did you deal with it?

Janet   Things hardly changed, mainly because of Karen's age. You see the boys were eighteen and sixteen. She was so self-sufficient. She would take herself off to Prince Charles every week for a blood test—I didn't go with her unless she wanted me to go for a drive with her—but she went there herself, and she rang for the results herself, and then if the counts were low and she had to start on the antibiotics then she'd do that herself. Because of her age, I think we didn't have to change anything.

We didn't give her all the attention—not that we were conscious of not doing it. But we didn't have to. We just didn't. We weren't conscious of giving the boys more attention, because they were just the same.

Probably Bruce and Gary at school—maybe they missed out a little bit because sometimes I wouldn't be home when they got home from school. But I thought they were old enough to come home on their own, anyway. I don't think things changed, do you Frank?

Frank   No.

Janet   Do you think they changed, Bruce?

Bruce Just a little bit. I thought I was left out there for a while, for three or four months.

Janet Did you?

Bruce I was left in the dark for a while. I didn't know what was going on.

Janet Did you think like that?

Bruce I thought you didn't care for me.

Janet Oh well, that wasn't right. We used to come home from hospital and we used to tell everybody all the results and what was going on.

Bruce I couldn't get a lot of information out of you, because it always upset you. We were never home, anyway. I was always up the hospital. Every afternoon, until about 10 o'clock at night, then I'd come home, and just go to school next morning.

Janet That was when she was in having treatment for the two or three days every three weeks.

Bruce And when she was in at the end.

Janet Oh, yes, when she was in Mount Olivet. That's a hospital for the terminally ill. That was a terrible time.

Frank Most people would come in and not come out. But it's a very good place.

Janet Their main aim is to keep them comfortable. Treat their pain and anxiety.

Mark Did you think of having her at home in the last stages?

Janet Yes, we did try. When things started to go bad ... they said there was nothing to help her, and she came home. She was here for two weeks, then she had six weeks in Mount Olivet.

Going back a little on that, in June or July they have the Terry Fox fun run here in Brisbane. It's to raise money for research into bone cancer. We all walked in that. We heard about it through the Queensland Cancer Fund and the teenage support group, which Karen really got involved in, so we all walked in that. She was starting to get the pain in her back, but she was still OK. A couple of Panadol would fix her for a couple of hours, so it wasn't too bad.

Then the kids all went in a bus to Seaworld. It had all been arranged. That was the Sunday. Then she was sore for a couple of days, but we didn't connect it with the cancer. We didn't think it had gone to another bone at all. We just didn't think of it. She was all right.

But then on the Wednesday morning she woke up and she was in really bad pain. She rang the ward— she was told always to ring the ward if she had a problem—and they told her to come in straight away. She was there for two weeks getting worse and worse really fast, and they had her on morphine tablets that were increasing in strength. They were supposed to last twelve hours, but they didn't, then she'd have to have a top up of morphine injection or mixture and that would make her sick. She got a lot weaker and much more pain in that time. They did a lot more tests, including a spinal one [a lumbar puncture]. They took some fluid out of her spine, and they found that there was Ewing's there in the spine.

When they told us the results, Karen and I were in the room. I can remember where the bed was exactly, and I remember where I was sitting. They came and told us that there was Ewing's in her spine. We looked at one another and we knew what that meant, because previously we'd been in to the Queensland Cancer Fund and learnt as much as we possibly could.

What we had read had been a real shock to us, but we were still OK because a lot of things didn't apply to Karen yet. We read where if there are secondaries, that decreases the chance of full recovery, and that was a shock. But it went on to say that if it recurred in another bone, the chances of recovery are slim. We thought: 'Wouldn't that be terrible', but we thought it didn't apply to Karen.

That's why when we were told these results, we knew.

But, you get over that shock because at that stage she was still alive and still OK, and they were treating her for pain, and ... you hang on to anything. I can't describe it. It's the lowest, lowest, lowest ... The bottom just falls out of everything. It's a feeling of disbelief. This is not happening to us. It happens to other people but not to us.

Anyway, she was there for two weeks and they were trying to get the pain under control and they did have it basically under control. Then they did more lung scans and Dr Hawson, the chief oncologist and two or three other doctors and the social worker—about eight people—came in to the room. I was there, and my father was there visiting, and Karen.

We just knew. We were waiting for the results all day. Dr Hawson had done his rounds and he'd left Karen till last. We were waiting for the results of the lung scan. When he came in, he stood at the end of the bed and he said: 'I don't know how to say this. I come into these rooms all the time, I give people bad news all the time, and I walk out, and that's my job. But ... there's no more treatment, the drugs were not working.'

By this time, Karen was starting to get confused about it all, and I was too. That's why we asked would Dr Hawson at some stage talk to all of us. All of our family went in and my parents and my sisters—that was when he told us that the change of drugs wasn't working.

Frank No, Karen told me first what was going to happen, then we went into the other room and all the doctors and others were there.

Janet That's right, I'm getting ahead of myself. They told Karen and I there was no more treatment and Karen asked: 'What does that mean, am I going to die?' and he said: 'Yes'. She asked: 'How long?', and he said: 'It could be weeks or months'. She had a bit of a cry, and so did I. That was a Friday.

Then he went on talking, and he stayed there for at least half an hour. Then a couple of them left, and when they all left, Karen was OK and I was OK—you find some sort of strength from somewhere—and then there's all these people you have to tell. So I rang Frank at work and got him to come to the hospital. And I got Gary from work and Bruce from school.

Bruce I wasn't at school at that time. I don't know where I was. I just took the day off. I don't know where I was. I was confused at the time. I didn't understand what was happening.

Janet I don't know, either. But I had to ring Gary at work. Karen said that she wanted to tell everyone herself, and she did. She told her best friend, Kym, and told everyone separately. I tried to protect her from it. I asked if I could do some of it. But she said: 'No, I want to do it.' She was incredibly brave.

Then there were things to organise. Dr Hawson asked if we could stay until Monday. He said he thought it was best if she went home and tried to get the most out of the rest of her life. He said there were a couple more drugs we could try, but they were in the experimental stages and if it was his daughter and his family, he wouldn't recommend it because they were so toxic. There would be no quality of life for her, and she would just be in hospital the whole time, because the drugs would just knock her around so much.

So this was the Friday and she wanted to get home straight away. But he talked her into staying until Monday so they could get the pain a bit more under control. To our surprise, the doctor came to visit her on Saturday and on Sunday. He didn't have to do that because it wasn't his weekend on. He wasn't on duty— you could tell by the clothes he was wearing that he wasn't on duty, but he just came in to see her. I thought it was really good of him to do that. He said telling her was one of the hardest things he'd ever had to do.

So on the Monday we came home by ambulance. That was a terrible trauma because she was in such pain. She was having morphine tablets and suppositories of something for pain. She was at home with us for about two weeks until we couldn't keep her here any longer—the pain was just increasing all the time. Mount Olivet Care was involved, nurses came every day and sometimes twice a day. They were available to us— we could ring them whenever we wanted, any time of the day or night. Somebody would come out and give her a morphine injection.

After a week here at home, when the slow release morphine tablets weren't working properly, they put a syringe driver in her chest and filled it with morphine and connected it to a pump. The strength of that had to be increased every day. With the increased strength of morphine she was getting more drowsy all the time.

Those two weeks were probably the worst two weeks for her because of the pain—we just couldn't get it under control. She had to tell us on a scale of 1 to 10 what she thought the pain was. She hated to do that— I think she just couldn't be bothered. But I tried to insist that she tell me because that was going to help them know what to administer.

But that two weeks was a bad time for her mentally as well as physically, because she definitely knew she was going to die. But she didn't know when, and we didn't know when.

She had her birthday, and it was Father's Day, and a few things like that. We put on a twentieth birthday for her here. We got a friend, Jenny McIvor from the Queensland Cancer Fund, to do the catering, and it was a really professional job. She was really sick that day—she couldn't have had a worse day than that. We didn't even know if she'd be able to be out here on the lounge. She was sick and vomiting and just terrible.

Those two weeks were terrible for her mentally. Being the type of person she was, she wanted to get everything organised. She wanted to tell the boys what she wanted them to have—she had a car, and a bike, a stereo system, things like that—and she talked to us all individually and she told us that she didn't want us to drop our bundles.

I felt terrible for her to have to do that, but since then people have said that that was what she wanted to do. It would have given her a lot of satisfaction. Getting organised would have given her a lot of peace of mind, so I don't feel quite so bad about it now. But it was a lot of mental suffering in that two weeks.

But then it got to the point where she couldn't get to the toilet and she needed a catheter and that couldn't be done at home. The doctor at Mount Olivet spoke to her one day and said: 'How about you come in to Mount Olivet for a while—it might only be for a week—until we get the pain under control.'

The only way they got her to go there was by saying it might only be for a week. She had a little cry that time. The only two times she cried were then and when she realised there was no more treatment.

The first week in Mount Olivet was awful because they decided to take her by ambulance every day to Royal Brisbane to give her radiation to the three different tumours that were in her spine. She was starting to go numb in her legs and that was really the reason they did that, to halt the tumour that was causing the numbness. With Karen the way she was, having been so active, being paralysed would have been one of the worst aspects for her.

They said it was only as a measure to help pain control. They did get feeling back in her legs, and she was so positive about it. A big group of doctors used to come and see her every day and she would just talk so much to them, she'd tell them how she was feeling. She was still so confident—not confident that she was going to live, she'd accepted that—but she was really strong. She'd accepted that she was going to die, but that was OK. I really think she thought that was OK.

She just wanted to oblige, to help people all the time, and to stop people getting morbid. The staff at Mount Olivet told us they learnt so much from having her there. They said normally a dying person does not think to tell them how they feel emotionally. The only thing they can normally get out of the average person who is dying is about the pain: is it better or is it worse? A yes or no answer. But she used to talk about everything.

Things got bad so fast that she couldn't move out of her bed. Then the increased morphine, I guess, dulled the senses.

Then she wanted someone there all the time. Then she went through a stage where she didn't want anyone close to her bed at all. She wanted us to push our chairs back. Someone there told us that that's often the way a dying person feels—they think everything is closing in on them.

I was there all the time. She didn't like to tell me, but the staff told me, that she wanted a bit of space without me being there. I obliged there, too, but that was hard.

Frank We really spent a lot of that last six weeks, and especially that last two weeks, there with her.

Janet She wanted her dog to come and see her up at the hospital. She wanted to get home. We'd always say we'd get the pain right, then see in a couple of days. Then a couple of days would pass, and the pain wouldn't be under control. Eventually she realised she wasn't going to get home, and she wanted her dog to come up.

They let us. That was upsetting. I mean it wasn't upsetting for her, but it was for me. I was afraid that when I left to take the dog home she'd be upset. At that stage the morphine was so strong—she'd started with 50 mg and was up to 400 mg in eight weeks or ten weeks.

Bruce I remember one night you weren't there and Dad wasn't there, I was looking after her, and I thought she was dying. Her breathing was getting slower and faster and slower and faster. I pressed the buzzer so many times, and nothing happened. I ran up the hallway trying to get a nurse, but there weren't many nurses around at that time.

Janet Yes, her breathing started to get worse in the last three weeks.

Bruce It just changed so quickly.

Janet But she went the whole week and didn't realise her breathing had changed because of the morphine. But then she was on oxygen, and she would just speak to us occasionally, and her right lung was absolutely full of tumours, so she had to lie on her right side to leave her left lung free to breathe.

Bruce She was on oxygen for the last week or so.

Mark Obviously you can't change what happened to Karen, but is there anything that has stuck in your mind that could have been done differently?

Janet I think the doctors did all they could. Karen's doctor, when she was first diagnosed, wasn't her doctor. He was overseas doing cancer research, and he told us that things wouldn't have been done any differently anywhere in the world. So we felt quite confident about that. I don't think the doctors at Prince Charles could have done any more and I don't think at Mount Olivet they could have done any better.

Frank That new drug they tried was an experiment.

Janet Yes, and she was also a guinea pig for a new anti-nausea drug, too. Ondansetron, it was.

Mark Did it help?

Janet Yes, it did.

Mark   Did you feel like you knew what was going on?

Janet   Yes, we did. Because she asked questions.

Frank   Then she explained to us everything that was happening.

Janet   One anxiety she had was how she was going to die, whether she would choke to death. She asked the doctor from Mount Olivet what form death would take. He assured her she would not choke to death. That was her great worry.

But she did have one anxious moment in that last week—she was in and out of sleep—when she opened her eyes and said 'Air, air.' That was the only time she ever complained about it. But within a minute she was back to sleep again.

You asked about if there was anything we would change if we could. There's one thing I do have the guilts about—I wasn't right there, touching her, holding her hand, when she died.

Frank   And I feel guilty because I didn't find it. Why didn't I find this thing before she got the secondaries? Obviously some cancers are very difficult to diagnose, but we were told it'd been there three years.

There's no way we would have known, but if we could have found it earlier then it's quite possible Karen would have lived another fifteen or twenty years. She may not have got it again.

Janet   You know, it's possible if she wasn't so fit we might have found it earlier or it might not have spread so quickly, but athletics was her life. Her whole life. And she'd done so much. She'd done more in her twenty years than many people do in a lifetime. She'd been overseas a couple of times, she'd been around the world through athletics.

I said to her a couple of times that I wished I could take her place. And I did. My children are not children any more. But she didn't like me thinking like that. She thought it was better for her to get it than me, because I had dependants. She said: 'I've done everything in life except get married and have kids', which she had.

So she was quite resigned to the fact. I wouldn't say she was happy to die, but she was resigned to the fact that she was dying. She accepted it.

Patrick McCabe

Interview with Patrick McCabe and his parents, Sue and Brian, at their Brisbane home. Patrick was born on 20 January 1976.

Sue   Patrick was about seven and a half. The first sign we had of it came when we went to Sydney on holidays in the Easter of 1983. He'd been playing over in the park, and he came back screaming. He had this sore chest. He wasn't just crying, he was screaming, screaming, screaming. It went on for a few hours.

So we took him up to the local hospital. They didn't know what was wrong with him, but they settled him down. They said we should go home and put a bag of frozen peas on his chest, which we did.

That seemed to settle him down for a while, but from that time, which was March or April, he kept having these recurrences of screaming. I took him to the doctor on several occasions. Patrick had had bad asthma—he'd been in and out of hospital a couple of times—and they put it down to muscle spasms and different things.

During that year we went to New Zealand, too—my mother was over there and quite ill—and I'd taken Patrick and my daughter. I don't think it happened over there, but.

Patrick   I can remember it happening down the road.

Sue   Yes. He used to scream and I just knew that it wasn't asthma, because asthma's not a painful thing. Anyway, we came to the October school holidays and I was pregnant with our third by this stage and we all went up to Bribie Island—the kids and my neighbour and her kids—and Patrick was coming out of the water and my friend Lorraine said: 'What's the matter with Patrick's chest? He's got a lump under his arm', and I said: 'Oh my God, he has, too'.

So we came home and Brian was home and Patrick was in the bath and I said to have a look at Patrick's chest. So next day I thought I'd better take him to the doctor and find out what it is.

Well, the doctor we'd been seeing was away and there was a locum there and he just took one look at it and said: 'I think you'd better go and have some X-rays taken.' So we had the X-rays taken and came back. It was the long weekend in October and that was on the Thursday. It was obvious there was a tumour there—a huge tumour.

Mark   Could you see it?

Sue   Oh, yes. They showed us the X-rays. It was the size of a football. It took his whole chest cavity. It had grown inward where a lot of them grow out first. It had grown into his chest cavity and when there was no more room for it to grow it was starting to come out.

On the Monday we had to go down to the hospital and we saw Dr Smith in the oncology unit down there. Patrick was in hospital that night, and they did a biopsy on the Wednesday morning. I think they told us what it was on the Thursday.

I knew it was something. I knew it wasn't just something trivial. But when they told us it what it was ... I was nearly six months pregnant at this stage so they were pretty careful how they told us. But it was something that you never ... you can't even

comprehend what it's like to be told something like
that.

Mark Before you were told, did you consider it might be
cancer?

Sue I think Brian did.

Brian It had to cross your mind.

Sue I think I thought it was, but I didn't really want to
think that it was. I thought: 'Yes, well, it could be
cancer, but he's only a little kid and kids don't get
cancer'. The thought had been there, but I hadn't
really seriously considered it, mainly because I didn't
want to.

Brian I can see the room now. They were examining
Patrick and they kept on making him move his arm
around in a large circular motion. They had a lot of
doctors in there and a couple of them had surprised
looks on their faces. To me, they couldn't understand
why Patrick didn't have any pain when he moved his
arm in a 360 degrees turn.

Then this other guy comes in and Smith was there,
the doctor who we got to know quite well, and they
were umming and aahing. I walked outside for a while
and came back in about ten minutes later, and it just
occurred to me. I said: 'Why are all these doctors here?
It must be something wrong.'

Then all these other doctors kept coming in. In the
end there must have been about twenty people in the
room—doctors and nurses and so on. I could see
Smith standing in a huddle in the corner with three
or four other doctors. The looks on their faces were
very serious.

It all connected. A whole group of doctors, a whole
group of nurses—it was like the whole club was in
there.

Sue Remember that was quite early. We had to get there
about 8:30 in the morning. Then the rest of that day
they took X-rays and we had to go over to the Holy

Spirit [Hospital] and they took CAT scans. I remember coming out of there, it was about 8:30 at night before we got back to the Children's Hospital, and they kept Patrick in. It was a horrible day.

Then Patrick had the biopsy on the Wednesday and they told us on the Thursday. Then they decided how they would treat it.

Mark   When they told you, did you understand what they were saying? Or did you just hear the word 'cancer' and block the rest out?

Sue   I understood it first time. They said to us it was one of two things—either a Ewing's sarcoma or a lymphoma. They said we would be a lot better off if it was a lymphoma.

Brian   We said: 'What do you think, Dr Smith?' I can remember him sitting there. He said: 'We hope it's a lymphoma' and I said: 'Why?' He said the treatment for lymphoma had advanced a lot more in the past two or three years than the treatment for Ewing's. I remember that distinctly.

Sue   By that stage, of course, we were hoping it was a lymphoma, then they told us it wasn't. They said his chances weren't real crash hot.

Mark   At that stage, did you know what was going on Patrick?

Patrick   I can't remember any of this.

Sue   They told Patrick exactly what was going on. After they told us, they said: 'Right, now we have to go and tell Patrick.' I think Brian and I wondered whether it was a good idea or not, but they were very insistent about it. They went up and told him that he was very sick, and . . .

Patrick   I can remember being told I was very sick, but I can't remember much else.

Sue   They told him what they were going to have to do. They told him he was going to have to have a lot of needles, and his hair was going to fall out. They went through it all.

Mark Do you think now that telling him was the right thing to do.

Sue Definitely. We were a bit worried, because we didn't know how he'd react.

Mark How did he react?

Sue I think it all went over the top of his head.

Brian I think we'd better tell him about why he doesn't remember much of this. Patrick, tell him about your memory, mate.

Patrick I can't remember much at all. It all seems blocked out.

Mark Is it that you can't remember much about being a kid? Or is it that you can't remember much about the cancer?

Patrick I can't remember much about the cancer. I can remember having it, but I can remember having needles and my hair falling out and going to school and stuff like that, but the details . . .

Mark So the treatment hasn't affected your memory.

Patrick No, I don't think so. It's just that I don't want to remember, because I can remember bits from before that, before I was sick.

Sue We'd been moved around a lot before we came here, and occasionally he might think of something from those times.

Brian I think it might be that some of the treatment he had, some of the chemotherapy, has deleted part of his memory.

Sue I don't know about that.

Patrick I can remember actually having chemotherapy. I can remember being in the little room at the back there, and the nurses and that. I can remember that.

Sue It's nothing like it is now. The Children's Hospital is nice and new and modern now. Where Patrick went it was at the back of haematology and it was the size of a bathroom and he had to sit on the floor. It was a matter almost of strapping them down to put a needle in—it was pretty horrific. It was really dreadful.

Mark So we're at the stage where you've been told what was going on, and they're deciding what the best form of treatment was. Did they talk to you about the options? Or did they just tell you what was going to happen?

Sue They just told us what was going to happen. They didn't tell us the options.

Brian Maybe there weren't any. Smith told us what he thought he should do. He told us they had a big meeting every week of everybody from all the hospitals where they looked after children with cancer. And sometimes he got an idea from someone else from another hospital, or someone in Melbourne had come up with another alternative, or of using a treatment that could be given in a slightly alternative way. I remember him quite specifically telling us about that.

Then he showed us the X-rays, and told us what was happening there. From what I recall he told us how they were going to approach the problem. He told us: 'This is they way we think he should be treated.' He didn't tell us: 'This is what we're going to do.'

Sue He told us what they had arrived at.

Brian He was talking as if we were a part of the decisions being made.

Sue He never ever spoke down to us, or spoke to us like we were idiots, like some doctors do.

Patrick Like you're a lower class of person.

Sue Smith was never like that. He would speak to you as if you understood, and if you didn't, he would go through it all again. So you knew exactly what was going on.

Anyway, because the tumour was so large, they couldn't operate straight away. They had to reduce it. So he had six weeks of chemotherapy and that reduced

it right down. They said if they could get it to the size
of an orange they could look at doing something about
it. And they did.

That was the end of October, and it was on the
nineteenth of December he had the operation to
remove it all.

Oh yes, and during it all they found secondaries on
his skull. You can still see where his hair doesn't grow
properly. He had massive doses of radiation to his
skull, and his hair has never grown.

Mark   It's halfway to a good haircut, isn't it?

Sue   Yes. Anyway they found secondaries about the size
of a five cent piece. Along the way they had said that
it was only in his chest, but they looked from top to
toe. And they said we had to understand that if they
found it somewhere else it would reduce his chances.
So when they said it was in his skull, we thought: 'Holy
shit!' That really brought us down.

But they continued with the chemotherapy, then
after he had the tumour removed he had radiation for
three weeks. They radiated that area, and it just
disappeared.

They removed the tumour, but unfortunately they
found it had already spread from the third rib into the
second and fourth ribs, so they had to take the three
ribs out. It had already attached itself to part of his
lung, so part of his lung had to come out. And all the
muscle and tissue it was attached to had to come out.
He lost quite a bit of muscle and tissue.

Patrick   Then I had chemo again. How long was that for?

Sue   For a total of about twelve months. During that time
he had radiation for about three weeks. He'd go for
the chemo every seven or ten days—it depended on
the blood count.

Brian   A couple of times they'd do the blood count and
we'd ring up and they'd say it was a bit low, we'd better
wait a couple of days. He had a really nice teacher at

the time—a bloke called Ken Swan. We had to go to school a few times to pick him up, and Ken would be really upset.

Sue The poor man. He'd see us coming and the whole expression on his face would change. He was really good because he had Patrick in grade 3 and they put Patrick in his class in grade 4 because he knew what was going on. He had the other kids pretty well sorted out, too.

He was tuned in. Not that he knew everything that was going on, but he made the effort. He had a good outlook on it, although you could see that it really upset him.

Mark You have two other children, both younger. How did you handle that?

Sue Well, I was pregnant with Laurence and Elizabeth was two and a half to three. That was fairly hard. I don't have any family here—Brian's mother is the only family. But I was very fortunate to have an excellent neighbour. We wouldn't have been able to survive without them because they were just terrific. Elizabeth could stay there the whole day, and some nights, and I didn't even have to ask.

She'd just stay there, and they'd take her out. They used to take her out to everything. We'd come home and they might have cooked tea for us.

It's people like that just . . . you can't describe what they do for you.

Mark How did Elizabeth cope with the disruption to her life?

Sue It was just the way it was. She didn't know any different. She was going to kindy a couple of days a week, and there were several times I had to get friends to pick her up from kindergarten. But I don't think she thought things were any different—she just thought that's the way things were. And because our neighbours were so great, she was perfectly happy with them.

Problems with the tape recorder meant this interview could not be transcribed fully.

Paul Price

Interview with Paul and Kathy Price in Wesley Hospital, Brisbane, on 6 December 1992. At the time of the interview, Paul was fairly weak and was having some difficulty speaking.

Paul   I first started to feel pain in about 1988. We had just come back to Brisbane and we had bought our own practice—we're both doctors—and I just ignored the back pain for several months. I finally had some X-rays done, and they were reported as normal.

We were waiting for Claire, and when she was born I made an appointment to see an orthopaedic surgeon. He could tell straight away the X-rays weren't normal. He sent me for a CAT scan and a bone scan. I can remember the radiologist still didn't think anything was wrong, but he came into the bone scan room and I was lying immobile. He came up to me and said: 'Dr Sugars was right, you know. There's something there.' I waited for about 20 minutes, panicking, and I thought that was really rough.

I was referred to Ian Dickinson and he told me I needed an operation, but first I needed chemotherapy, which Geoff Beadle did. I went through four months of chemo then had my surgery. It was pretty long surgery because the tumour was in my pelvis. I was very frightened the night before. I thought I was going to die, which wasn't giving much credit to the surgeon.

Anyway, I got over the surgery but couldn't walk for

about nine months after that. I had radiotherapy after the surgery. Then I had to get away because I was sick of the sight of doctors. Weren't we?

Kathy We sure were.

Paul We had a holiday, and then I came back to undertake chemotherapy, which lasted about eighteen months. It got that way that I would vomit, sometimes on the way to hospital, but I would vomit in anticipation of the chemo, which I found really hard to take. There was many a time I felt like quitting, but you wouldn't let me, would you?

Kathy No, not at that time.

Paul Kathy found that a little bit hard to take because she's got a vomit phobia and it was pretty hard to have a husband who, every six weeks, was going to vomit a lot.

Kathy It was very hard on the children.

Mark Would it start before the chemo?

Paul I'd start to feel sick the night before, and I'd have sedatives to help me sleep and try to get rid of the feeling. Then I'd take them the next morning, and by the time I had all that on board I'd be really sleepy.

Originally I could control the nausea until I got to the hospital, and I wouldn't start vomiting until I got into hospital, but I lost it a couple of times outside and in the car. I tried to take more sedatives once I got to the hospital, but that didn't work.

Kathy He saw a psychologist to try to help with that because it was getting so bad. It was getting to the stage where he wouldn't have been able to continue treatment unless something happened to change it. He had some behaviour modification to try to bring it under control, and that did stop it getting worse. It didn't improve it, but it stopped it getting worse. Then he had more sedatives.

So he was a bit bombed out, sometimes to the point where he wasn't really aware of what was going on.

That made it hard to actually get Paul into the hospital because he was still having trouble walking. He was using a stick some of the time. So being under sedation, and vomiting at the same time, even in the lift . . . the practicalities of it were very difficult.

Paul started off just staying one night in hospital, but the vomiting was so prolonged he ended up staying two nights just to try to get him going a bit better by the time he came home. But he still felt unwell for a week after each treatment.

Paul   That's right. I'd feel nauseated and washed out. The thing was that once I got over that, I'd have a week in which my blood count was dropping and I'd feel lousy from that. I think coping with the chemotherapy was the hardest part.

Kathy   During that time Paul went back to work. He'd have three weeks where he was under the weather from the chemotherapy, then three weeks where he was reasonably well. So he got a job where they allowed him to work for those three weeks. He did that for months.

Mark   Did you find ways of handling the chemo?

Kathy   Counting down to how many were left.

Paul   Yes, that was the only thing that kept me going.

Kathy   And the hope that maybe it was going to be worthwhile. The hope that maybe it would cure him. And also the thought that if Paul did exactly what the doctors said to do, and had exactly as many treatments as they said, and still got a recurrence, well at least we had done whatever was possible. But if he'd bailed out early, we might be left thinking 'if he'd just had one more treatment, it might have worked'. As it's turned out, it probably wasn't all that helpful, but . . .

Mark   Do you regret now having eighteen months of chemo?

Kathy   The second lot was eighteen months.

Paul   Oh, no. I can see the benefit it had in that it kept the tumour at bay for that time, where I probably would have had the recurrence sooner. I don't regret that decision. I guess I can say I've stuck it out.

Kathy It was only about three months after Paul finished the chemo that there was the first sign of the recurrence. It was a spot on his chest X-ray, which his doctor said wasn't anything, because it was too small.

But many chest X-rays later, it became obvious that there were more of them and that definitely they were secondaries. So then came the next treatment, which was radiotherapy. Initially it was thought there was to be no more treatment. That was it. But then Bernie Mason decided it was worth giving this a try, even though it's rarely done. The actual radiotherapy wasn't too bad, but the problem was the shortness of breath afterwards as a side effect.

Paul We went along fine until August this year, then on 19 August I collapsed at home. It was a stroke from secondaries in my brain, which apparently are as rare as anything. But the longer you live, the more you get a chance of rare things going wrong.

I was rushed in here, then the neurosurgeon took me over to Royal Brisbane, and operated, then brought me back here. I went over there again for a second operation, to clean out some tumour on the other side. I spent eight and a half weeks in hospital. I recovered pretty well. I had total brain radiotherapy after that, because the tumour has been sensitive to irradiation.

There was much discussion about whether I should have the treatment. This sounds like putting the cart before the horse, but I tolerated it very well therefore I thought it was worth having.

Mark Kathy, do you feel you've been informed of everything that's happened along the way.

Kathy Not all the time, even though we're doctors.

In the beginning, we were informed of everything, even to the extent that when Paul first had the X-rays, well ... The worst thing as far as I'm concerned was that we were sitting outside the X-ray director's office waiting to take the X-rays back to see the specialist and he came out to me and said: 'You're a doctor, aren't you?' and I said 'Yes' and he said 'Come in, I want to show you something'. I said 'Can Paul come too?' and he said 'No, just you'.

I went in and he had the CAT scans and pictures up on the X-ray box. Even someone who wasn't a doctor could have seen the size and the extent of the tumour. He just stood me there in front of these things, saying 'It's obviously malignant and it's really bad'. Then he sent me outside to sit with Paul. Even in those early days we had made a decision to be open with each other, and I told him there was something fairly bad there.

We were told everything about how bad the surgery was going to be. I think we were sometimes told that it was going to be worse than it actually was. It was only recently with the decisions on whether to continue treatment or not that sometimes, maybe, the doctors have been making a few decisions that we weren't really aware of. In retrospect, it would have been better if we had been able to talk about it openly.

Mark What sort of things?

Kathy Well, Paul's now got a three to four centimetre secondary in his lungs which has recurred despite the radiotherapy. The doctor felt maybe Paul had had enough treatment. Certainly that's how I've been feeling, because it's been such a long and stressful time. Having been through all the time with Paul and his stroke and everything else, I guess I came to that conclusion a little earlier than Paul did. That it was time that we shouldn't be doing any more treatment. Sometimes you have to say enough's enough. And even though that's very hard to do, that was how I'd come to feel.

Paul hadn't reached that decision yet, but the doctor also thought that was the right decision. Therefore he didn't offer Paul treatment for this secondary when he found it, but sort of fobbed us off. But then when Paul said that he wanted treatment, the doctor said he was prepared to go ahead with it. He's now told us that he knew it was a secondary all along but he didn't want to offer Paul more treatment, because he felt it was just getting too much.

I feel that in that sort of situation, it's really important that doctors are honest with patients. It may make it a more difficult decision for people, but you need to have all the facts about all the problems that may be arising from treatment. It worries me that as doctors we had a lot more knowledge than the average person, but sometimes we still didn't feel we knew what was going on. Sometimes that's for the best, I guess, but there's a fine line between talking too much and not talking enough.

Mark Have you been treated as a partner, or as a doctor?

Kathy A bit of both. Even if I haven't been treated as a doctor, sometimes I needed to react as a doctor because that's what I know how to do in the hospital situation. But it's hard separating the roles.

When Paul was at home that last weekend, I didn't know what to do. I knew as a wife what to do, and I knew as a doctor what to do, but I didn't know which one to be. As a wife I would have known that the thing to do was to ring the doctor straight away and tell him things weren't right, but as a doctor I didn't know how far I should go before ringing somebody in case they might just think I was being silly. It's very difficult to know how to react.

And certainly after Paul had the stroke, I was treated as nothing. Not here [at Wesley Hospital], but I think that's what happens to relatives in general, particularly in neurosurgery. They tend to be left out in the waiting room, waiting to hear, and not knowing what's going on, even to the extent that when Paul was transferred to one of the wards, I was left outside with nobody bothering to tell me he'd gone. There was a great lack of communication. I was there in a highly stressed state because Paul had had a very life-threatening thing happen to him and at that time his personality was really ... a little bit different. It was very difficult at that stage because of what had happened to his brain, and there were all these major things happening to him, and he'd had a stroke, he couldn't move his side, and he couldn't talk, yet there was very little communication happening. I just felt I was left out in the cold. I was the person doing all the worrying, but I didn't know what was happening. And if I felt like that as a doctor, how would the average person feel?

So sometimes it's been harder being a doctor. Sometimes the more facts you have, the more you worry.

Paul Because we're doctors, we have more of an insight into what goes on. I don't think that helps. I think I'd rather be ignorant than have knowledge of my condition.

Kathy Whereas I feel differently. I feel I would rather know what's going on. Like with this present problem he's having with his abdomen, I'd be happy for Paul to have a CAT scan to know what's causing his problems. Is it a tumour in his abdomen or not? Because then we'd know, rather than thinking that maybe it is, or maybe it isn't. So then if we had a test that showed it wasn't, we'd know.

But Paul and the doctor both feel it's better not to know, because if there's a tumour there they're not going to do anything about it. So rather than knowing the tumour was there and doing nothing, they'd rather not know at all. I guess that's just different opinions of the same situation.

One important thing. When Paul was first admitted for chemo, and the nurse was doing the admission, and I was sitting there breastfeeding this little three and a half week old baby, she was asking all these questions and then she said to us: 'And this wouldn't have made any difference to your life?' It was just the most amazing thing. I just burst into tears. She hadn't realised what she'd said. Here's this young man who, up until three days before, had been working full-time as a GP with two little children, and a whole future to look forward to, as anybody else in that situation would, then suddenly to be confronted with this, and for her to say such an inane thing, it was just devastating. It's never got out of my mind that somebody could actually think that.

Since then most people have been very caring, but to think that that one person could have that bad attitude was really distressing. It wouldn't have mattered whether I was a doctor or a streetsweeper— it would still have been terrible to hear such an attitude.

I suppose having children of any age makes it all the more difficult.

Mark How old are they?

Kathy Claire's nearly four and Richard's six. Richard does not remember a time before Paul was sick, because he was only two and a half when Paul was diagnosed, and all he knows is life with a Dad who's sick, with a Dad who can't run, and with a Dad who can't do rough 'n' tumble things with him because it might hurt. It's been tough, especially in recent times, because we can't plan to do anything. Whenever we book somewhere Paul gets sick again and we don't do it. We make promises that don't come to fruition. And his Dad's been in hospital for such a long time. It's been very distressing.

But on the other hand, the positive side of it is that

a lot of the time Paul has been home and reasonably well. He's been able to go to the school and do a lot of things that fathers don't normally get to do. And go to kindy roster, and do things like that. So there's been those positive things, too.

Mark You probably know more about your kids than the average father.

Paul Yes, I'd like to think so. It's been an enormous strain on Kathy and the kids, and the kids react in different ways. Claire's OK—perhaps she's too young to understand. But Richard refuses to come and visit me in hospital, because he doesn't like hospitals. He's OK at home when I'm at home, but as soon as I come back into hospital he refuses to come up and see me. He's got a thing about vomiting.

Kathy He's beome quite fearful of the whole thing, especially the vomiting part of it. Because when Paul had the stroke, the children were there and they saw him being carried out of the house vomiting. That's the image he had of his father. The thought of him coming home terrified Richard—he thought we would run out of vomit buckets for his father. Obviously it had been blown out of all proportion to him, but that's what he associated with his father.

Paul Then he refused to talk to me on the telephone, because he thought I might vomit down the telephone.

Kathy Then once I explained to him that Paul couldn't vomit down the telephone, he said he didn't want to talk because he was frightened he wouldn't understand him on the phone. So eventually we got over that, and he's talked to Paul twice on the phone now. It's very distressing to Paul to be this ill and his son doesn't even want to talk to him on the phone. It's a very distressing thing for Paul to hear me say: 'Come and talk to your father on the phone' and to hear him say: 'No, I don't want to.' It's a very difficult thing to be rejected.

In fact, through this whole thing Paul's had to cope with a lot of rejection, especially by Claire. He looked after her a lot, because I had to go back to work when she was only five weeks old, and up until she was five months old he looked after her more than I did.

When Paul had to come in for surgery, Claire was about five months old. Even though we came up to see him, she just completely forgot him. And even for months after that, she wouldn't even take a bottle from him. She'd just scream if he touched her, and it was only very gradually that she came to accept him. That's been very hard to accept.

But I guess to a little tiny baby, he just didn't look like the same person. He was wearing hospital gowns, and he was really pale because he'd lost so much blood. During the operations he needed 25 bags of blood, and he just didn't look the same. It was just one of those things that took a long time to get over. It was very stressful.

But now Claire's really keen to come up and see Paul, because she actually likes hospitals. And she's always keen to talk to him on the phone. They react totally differently. When Paul's in hospital, Richard's really withdrawn and obviously quite stressed by it, yet Claire wants to come up to the hospital and is really caring.

Then when Paul comes home, Claire starts throwing tantrums again. But I guess she's just used to coming to hospital. It's part of life.

Paul It's very hard on Kathy, too. She's suddenly had to take on so many roles that up until I had that stroke were mine. She's got to look after the pool, and the gardens, and cooking, and she does a lot at home, which is not fair on her. But she's got to do it.

Mark How have you managed financially?

Kathy I've actually worked more than I wanted to because, foolishly or not, we tried to be optimistic. In the time between when Paul finished his chemo and he developed the secondaries, we took on a job we thought would be good for us. It had always been our dream that we would have our own practice together because we really liked working together. That's what we were doing when Paul was diagnosed. So we knew we couldn't start a practice together, because that was foolish, so we took on a job together. We thought that was the next best thing.

Then when Paul got sick again, that meant that I had to do all the work, which was really silly. But on the other hand, if it had turned out that Paul was cured and everything was fine, it was the right thing to do. We took a gamble, and it didn't come off. But now I've given up that job and I'm working part time in another job which is easier.

I have to realise that until Claire finishes high school, I'm going to be depended on for the after school hours. And if I'm working in a job like I was then, with long hours, then that's really impractical.

It's been hard for me because I've now left two jobs that I really liked, and was really happy with, because of Paul. It's been hard to leave something I was happy in because of something that was out of Paul's control, but that's just the way it worked out.

Paul had disability insurance, which we can't speak highly enough of. It's been such a boon. And he also has life insurance, which ... which ... maybe it's because we were so prepared that this has happened to us. Most of our friends can't say they had private health insurance, life insurance and disability insurance, and yet we were the ones who had to use it. Maybe it was because we were too practical and too prepared that this has happened.

But part of the reason I have kept on working through all of this is that I know of the possibility, the very strong possibility, that I'm going to have to be the breadwinner. And I have to keep being able to do it. Because once we don't have the disability insurance, because it isn't paying any more, then I'll have to work to be the breadwinner. We're anticipating the life insurance money, but I'll have to keep working.

It also helps to just get out and be different, to be myself, not to have to worry about someone else's problems for a while. I can just blank out. That helps. I can talk to different people and not be tied up in my own problems all the time. So I have kept on working and so financially, it hasn't been a strain. Although it ended up we had to move house, mainly because the house we were living in was a two storey house and Paul couldn't get up to the bedroom. He used to sleep in the rumpus room. We decided that the steps were a real drag for him, even when he could walk up and down them. So we decided to move closer to my parents, who have done everything for us.

Mark On another track, you said that at one stage you thought there was a chance of a cure. Can you tell me more about that?

Paul From day one, I had this optimism that I would be cured. Until a few months ago, I was still fairly optimistic that I would be a long-term survivor. It was probably not very realistic, but I've always had this feeling that I could survive the cancer.

There wasn't any doubt about the diagnosis, and it was pretty devastating to find out I had a bone tumour. But there always seemed to be something that could be done. Now there isn't. Each stage that we went through—the initial chemotherapy, surgery, radio-therapy, then the second lot of chemo—seemed to be allowing for a potential cure.

I guess Geoff Beadle was rather pessimistic, or maybe realistic, but particularly the orthopaedic surgeon felt that with combination treatment the odds of survival were 75 per cent. Geoff Beadle thought at best they were 50 per cent. But I hung my hat on the fact that I'd be in the right sub-set of the statistics.

Kathy I thought that when Paul was first diagnosed, we knew older people who had cancer. And they'd say: 'Why me, why me?' I was angry with them, because I used to think: 'It's OK for them, they're old, but Paul's only young.'

But I've realised that it doesn't matter how old you are—it's just as hard to cope with. It's really, really hard. It's not so much the disease that is hard, it's the treatment. Paul wasn't sick except for the treatment. There's been very little of this that's caused Paul any pain or suffering that hasn't been from the treatment, until the stroke. Sometimes it's been hard to believe that that's what was wrong, because it didn't seem to affect him too much. It was the treatment that caused him to be sicker. But now it's the disease.

Mark At some stage you changed your mind and started thinking that a cure was not realistic. What happened?

Paul Probably when I got the secondaries in my lungs. The first thing that happened was it came back in my rib, which was painful. Then they found the secondaries in my lungs. I then realised that cure was probably not realistic, and the best I could hope for was long-term survival, whatever that means.

Mark What did you mean by it?

Paul Five years. I've always said that I wanted to get to my ten year reunion, which is next year. I can't guarantee that I'll make it. I guess I had five years, or more than five years, in mind.

Kathy We were told there was some sort of cut-off—if you survive five years you survive long term. But I guess that five years is close to being up with Paul, but it doesn't look like he's going to survive.

Mark Have you found a lot of support from friends? I

meant both physical and emotional support. Or have they tended to leave you alone?

Paul Friends rally around at points of crisis, then they tend to forget for a while.

Kathy They don't forget, but they go from ringing very frequently to not ringing very frequently. And then you get to the point where when something serious has gone wrong, you just can't face ringing the whole circle of friends and letting them know. I'm sure thay're all thinking about us, but they just don't ring as often.

Paul They've got their lives to lead, and you can understand it. They haven't got time to get too involved with us. I don't resent that.

Kathy We've been lucky that my parents live so close and have retired, and have been willing to do whatever they have been able to do for us. It's one of those situations where if we didn't have them, we would call on other people. But because Mum and Dad are there and available, and people know that, then we tend to ask Mum and Dad all the time. Every time Paul needs to go to hospital we just get in touch with them and they look after the kids. Or if something goes wrong, then they're there.

It's one of the situations where it's always easier to ask a relation, than a friend.

Paul We're really grateful to Kathy's Mum and Dad. I'm sure we wouldn't have got this far without them.

Mark Is there anything that you can think of that could have been handled differently? Are there things that you would change now if you could, apart from the outcome?

Kathy I guess the big thing is that we should have acted on Paul's pain sooner. To us, it was just a normal back pain like anybody else has. It was just the same as back pain that I get—it just turned out to be different.

But in retrospect, even if we'd done something sooner, the X-rays would still have been reported as normal. So things wouldn't have changed all that much. It wasn't until Paul's pain was very bad that he decided to go see a specialist. So we couldn't have changed that, anyway. But you still always think that if Paul had been treated sooner, he would have had a better chance.

The other thing is that we had only tried traditional forms of treatment. We avoided alternative forms of treatment, except that Paul was doing transcendental meditation for a while, although that was more for relaxation rather than for any effort to cure the disease. Even though the traditional medicine has been so horrible, it's still the only thing we had any faith in.

Also, we should have upgraded our health insurance to keep more in touch with what the hospital fees are. We should have upgraded to the highest level you could get, where we only upgraded to the second highest level.

Another regret I have is that we didn't get a video camera and tape Paul while he was still all right and active. For me to tape Paul as he is now, well, it isn't the memory we should be leaving for the children. We want them to remember him the way he used to be.

He's writing a diary for the children. I think it's important for people in this situation to leave something behind for the children. Not just the last five minutes, but to start earlier and write down their thoughts and feelings on the world. And tell them what used to happen, and what their childhood was like. To help him, Bernie Mason has loaned him his computer so he can work on it. So they can have a memory of him. Even though the children will remember something, they won't necessarily remember the good times.

The other thing is that we should not have been so practical. When Paul was well, we should have enjoyed life more, because now it's too late.

Mark Is there anything you think is important that we haven't talked about?

Paul I'd just like to acknowledge my wife. She's been a wonderful support for me through these three or four years, and I wouldn't have been able to survive for as long as I have without her.

Paul died at Mount Olivet Hospital on 23 February 1993.

Sam Sciacca

Interview with Con and Tina Sciacca, parents of Sam and Zina, in their Brisbane home. Sam was born on 12 March 1973, and died on 13 April 1992 at the age of 19.

Con He first started getting symptoms of the disease in about April 1991, when he was complaining of a sore back. We took him to the GP who referred us to a specialist, and they took X-rays, but nothing showed up.

From April through to 21 September 1991, when he was diagnosed, he showed from time to time that he had some pains in his back. We were told by the GP that in all probability it was just growing pains, because he was growing very quickly. He seemed to grow very tall very quick. From the age of about sixteen and a half to seventeen and a half he seemed to just sprout. I'm talking anything up to five or six inches in a year. It was incredible. We were told that it was possibly just growing pains.

I do remember, though, that his pains were getting worse. Around about June or July he started limping a bit. We just put it down to the growing pains. A couple of times I distinctly remember Sam getting out of bed and saying: 'Oh, Dad, this back's killing me' and I'd go to his bedroom and massage it where it was hurting him, around the region of his lower back on the left hand side. It seemed to give him a bit of relief. I remember him saying: 'Thanks, Dad, I really appreciate that' and I ended up going to sleep in his bed with him.

Then you could still see him limping. You couldn't see a lump, though, because he was fairly ... he was fairly ... he was overweight, and he had big rolls of fat there. If he was real skinny you probably could have seen it.

But it wasn't until about 20 September I came home one night, it was a Thursday night, and he was sitting on the chair. I said to him: 'Son, what's wrong', and he said: 'I don't know Dad, this back's killing me'.

I instinctively went for his forehead and said: 'You've got a fever, mate, you've got a fever', and we called out Dr Rosendahl, my friend and GP, and he came around and took some tests and so forth. The very next night I was attending a function at the Italian-Australian Centre for some United Nations thing, and my wife rang me to say that Dr Rosendahl had rung up to say there were abnormalities found in Sammy's blood and we had to take him to the hospital immediately.

That Friday night we took him to the Wesley Hospital here in Brisbane and put him under CAT scans and everything. He had tests night and morning and night, and they found that he had cancer. We also gave him the MRI as well, the magnetic resonance imaging. We did the lot.

Then a couple of days later, the orthopaedic specialist operated and found that it was indeed cancer. A couple of days later they diagnosed it for sure as being Ewing's sarcoma of the bone, starting in the pelvis and with a number of metastases. There was one on his cheek, one on his left knee and one in his left arm.

We treated him with the normal chemotherapy. Dr

Geoff Beadle told us that if the chemotherapy didn't work—we treated it very aggressively—that if it didn't work he'd be flat out lasting a couple of weeks.

But it did work, for a while of course, then the usual story. It became resistant to it. There was a little bit of an increase in the tumour about a month after the original chemotherapy treatment, but he was OK for two or three months. We had him on alternative therapies, we had him on a number of things. Anyway, I'll let you ask the questions.

Mark   What else did you try?

Con   There's a fellow who's very well known here by the name of Dr Henry Oseiki. He's not a doctor, he's a nutritionist. His wife Vera is a medical practitioner. We had him on intravenous vitamin C, plus a vitamin regimen as well. We tried all of that. He seemed to feel better after he'd had his vitamin C, but one can't be sure. But certainly his white cell count bounced back pretty quick—the vitamin C must have been helping that. And with the massive dose of chemotherapy he was getting, one would have thought it was killing them completely.

But the funny thing is he hardly ever got an infection, even with all the chemotherapy. I do believe that the alternative therapy helped him. My doctors had no problems with Sam having that as an adjunctive treatment to counteract the debilitating effects of the chemotherapy.

Mark   You weren't looking for alternative treatments instead of the traditional?

Con   I looked at everything. If I could have found anything which I could have believed in and which I thought would have given us some chance, I would have just put him on that.

But it was pretty obvious that he was so far gone that my specialists told me that if I was not giving him the chemo, I was virtually stuffing him up altogether. That he had no chance, and the cancer would just keep travelling.

And for a while, the chemotherapy was working. It was inhibiting the growth. There was a slight decrease in the tumour size, then eventually it was pretty obvious that if we gave him any more chemo it would kill him outright, so we stopped chemo about two months before he died. He went downhill very rapidly after that.

We also tried another treatment. Some cousins of mine knew a cancer specialist in Italy at Bologna. I went there in January and took the family over. We went for a double purpose—faith healing at a place called Banneau in France, which is a shrine where the Blessed Mother of God is said to have appeared. We're Catholics. There's a shrine there to her—documented miracles and that sort of stuff. We went there and we also went to Lourdes in France. We went and saw the Pope and had a private audience with him. We actually had Mass in his private chapel.

Mark Did you go there blindly reaching for anything, or were you really believing this would help?

Con The way Tina and I figured it was this. According to the statistics we had seen, Ewing's sarcoma is enormously rare, about one in 500,000. I had read that documented cases of unexplained medical miracles have happened. In Lourdes, in France, supposedly one in 40,000 get miraculously cured. That's documented. They have hospitals there that document these things, and you can't get through this unless there is absolutely no medical reason for these miraculous cures. I know of people who first went there in 1972. They took the body bag with them, and he's still alive.

So I figured if one in 40,000 can get cured, and he's one in 500,000 that gets it . . .

You've got to understand. When you're a parent, it doesn't matter that he was our only son, but when you're a parent, you'll do anything. Even if it's a one in a million chance, even if it's one in 100 million, you've got to do something. You can't just sit back and let it happen, and not think you did everything. So I went there never really expecting that he was going to be cured, and maybe that's why we didn't get the miracle, but I went there hoping that maybe, just maybe, and it doesn't matter how small that maybe was, that just maybe that it would work.

We went to a place in the province of Puglia in southern Italy called San Giovanni Ritondo, which is a place where a holy man by the name of Padre Pio is supposed to have lived and helped with myriads of miracles. We actually prayed at his tomb.

We did the religious thing, the faith thing. We tried that. We tried the medical, the traditional. We tried the adjunctive treatment through vitamin C and vitamins. We took him to things that I would never have believed in my life I would have gone to. We went to healing masses with the charismatic renewal movement of the Catholic Church. I actually went to one of those visiting priests at the Sydney Hordern Pavilion and took Sam down there, only a week before he was paralysed when the cancer travelled up to the top of his spine. We took him there and we went through the praising God and all that. We did it all.

In addition to that, we even tried this professor at Bologna who gave us treatment with some stuff called Sandostatin. Dr Geoff Beadle can tell you, because we checked with him that none of this stuff we were going to inject into Sam was going to kill him even earlier than he was going to die. We gave him injections for two months of this treatment given to us by this professor, a little old professor who looked like Einstein. He's one of these sorts of blokes who, according to the promotion we received from friends and relatives in Italy, he had cured people with cancer. Using medicine, but not traditional medicine. The point was that it was just another avenue available to us, and we wanted to try it.

We took Sam to Italy in late January/early February, we went all the way to Bologna and we put him on this treatment. This treatment was very expensive, it cost us thousands, but it didn't matter. I haven't got a lot of dough—it might look like I have but I haven't—but money wasn't a problem. It never arose, but if it was a question of money, then I'd have gone and robbed a bank if I had to. I wouldn't have minded doing fifty years in gaol if I could have let him live.

We tried everything. Most people do that. I'm fortunate, because I've got a lot of influence and I can go and see people like the Pope and at least that gives us some inner peace. I mean the Pope blessed him— put his hand on Sam's head and blessed him personally. It was just great. Sam wasn't really religious, I wasn't really religious either. I never even used to go to church, although I do now, I go almost every day.

But the point is that we tried everything we could try. At the end we were really getting desperate. We'd heard somewhere that paw paw juice, treated a certain way, can stop the multiplication of the cancer cells. So we had our next door neighbours getting paw paw leaves and boiling them in accordance with this recipe by this woman who has done it for years and kept her cancer under control. Sammy was drinking this stuff until two days before he died.

We tried every bloody thing. We didn't just sit back and say: 'Well, Sammy's going to die'. We didn't just accept it.

We never told him. He never knew that he was dying. He never knew that he was dying. It may have dawned on him towards the end.

Mark You didn't tell him, or he didn't know? Do you genuinely think he didn't know?

Con   I genuinely think he may have known in his heart, but he didn't want to accept it. He was too young. He used to say to me: 'Dad, I don't want to die. I'm only eighteen. Why should I get this?' At that age, I don't think kids even have any concept of death.

The answer to your question is that we never told him, because we figured that if we'd have told him: 'Sammy, you're going to die', he'd have given up the ghost. But he never stopped fighting it, until the last fourteen hours.

He died at home at approximately 8.30 p.m. on Monday 13 April and that morning at about 5 a.m., we went to sleep, what sort of sleep you can have, and my daughter Zina and his cousin Robert stayed with him in his room, because he was paralysed from the beginning of February right through to when he died, because the cancer had travelled up his spine and lodged in the third or fourth vertebra. He didn't lose weight, he didn't waste away, but the cancer travelled through his skin, and he had bumps on his head, and the last day it actually travelled to his eyes.

But this particular morning my daughter came running in at about 5 a.m. saying: 'Dad, Dad, Sammy's babbling. He's talking but he's not making any sense. And his right eye's closed up.' There'd been nothing wrong with his eyes before that.

So I went running in and Sam's trying to lift himself up. His left arm was almost wasted away from the cancer. He was trying to reach up to the handle, like they have above a hospital bed, and he was so frustrated, he was always trying to move. And he's saying: 'Come on Dad, come on Dad, let's try, let's do it Dad, let's do it'. He was still fighting. He raised himself—don't ask me how—he raised himself off the bed in a superhuman effort.

So, I don't know. There's no doubt he knew he was in deep shit. He knew he was in deep shit. But I don't really believe that he wanted to think about it. Sam was a fighter. There was just no way he was going to think that this was going to get him. I don't know if that's answered your question, but we'd like to think that he didn't know.

Sam was the sort of bloke who never wanted to face bad things. He was a gentle kid. He didn't like drama or fighting or that sort of stuff. I think that even though he knew deep down, he just didn't want to know about it. He just figured that knowing about it was silly. I used to say rosaries with him every night and we used to say some prayers. He'd say: 'Dad, let's say some prayers' on the basis that we might be able to heal him through faith.

But I'm convinced, by things he'd say, that he never knew how bad he was. He'd say: 'You know Dad, I seem to be getting worse instead of better', and if he knew he was terminal, he wouldn't be expecting to get better.

Mark Was he a fairly young eighteen or old eighteen?

Con I'd say he was a youngish eighteen. He was a real homebod. He didn't get into strife and he wasn't going out all the time. All his friends were always coming home to my place. They still come here all the time, we're all close. They all enjoyed coming home and seeing Sam at home. During his sickness they were there all the time, all the time. They were always visiting him. They were all there with him the night he died. They were all there with him. He took his last breath and we were all there with him. Incredible.

Mark Was he glad to have a lot of people around?

Con He liked to have his friends around. He didn't like to have people around that he hardly ever saw. We kept anyone who hardly ever saw him away. We just didn't see the point. If anyone who didn't see him much

wanted to come, we'd tell them not to. We thought
that he'd think there was something wrong if all these
people that he hadn't seen for years started turning up
to see him.

But he enjoyed the company of his own friends. He
was still pretty chirpy. He still had a pretty good sense
of humour. The blue nurses would come and we'd
change him and he'd get a bit dirty [irritable] because
the pain was killing him when we'd move him. We used
to move him from his bedroom to the kitchen/dining
room area. We'd need three or four of us because he
was so big and heavy. We'd put him in a wheelchair—
one would get his legs, one would get his arms. But
the last week or so it started getting really painful for
him and the last night, just travelling the thirty feet
from his bedroom, it killed him.

But up to the Sunday night—he died on the Monday
night—we still moved him.

Mark Was he glad to be at home?

Con Oh, mate, he didn't want to be at the hospital. He
was a homebod. He was very comfortable at home. On
the Thursday night before he died, Cliff Rosendahl
came to see him because he had so much pain. We
had him sitting up in one of the big lounge chairs.
He'd had about three blood transfusions during the
week because the cancer was just going wild. Cliff
looked at him and said: 'I've got to talk to your Dad'.
And he looked up at Dr Rosendahl and said: 'Why?
Can't you say it in front of me?' He was pretty well on
the ball. Dr Rosendahl said: 'All right Sam, all right. I
think you should go to hospital', because he knew he
was dying and only had a few days.

But Sam looked up at me with his sad eyes and he
said: 'Dad, I don't want to go to hospital' and I said:
'Don't worry son, you're not going to hospital'. He
hated the hospital, he hated it. We used to keep him
out of there as much as we could. Most of the time he

was sick he spent at home. He only went in for chemotherapy treatments. He had an operation to remove the cancer off the top of his spine. The doctor got it out without any damage to his spine, but it didn't make a lot of difference.

Then once he lost the feeling in his legs he was in real trouble. He got really upset about that, then gradually he lost it all. It was frightening stuff for him. So he suffered a lot, the poor kid, he suffered a lot.

You just can't understand why. People die, and people get cancer, but this bloody Ewing's sarcoma ... You're ducko. From the moment you've got it, you're ducko. You haven't got a hope.

The most difficult part I found was that you really couldn't do anything. You couldn't even put your mind at rest. If I could have got hold of something like we're doing now and been able to read it, and thought: 'Crikey, he's got metastases, and he's got it in the pelvis, there's been other kids that've had this and they've gone running round the whole world and put themselves into hock, and it's done nothing.' I mean if I could have seen that, we may have made better use of the time that we had. I don't know. Probably not— I don't think we'd have ever given up. I was pretty fatalistic about it, but my wife and daughter just refused to accept it. They said: 'If and when he ever dies, we'll mourn him then, not now.' That was a great attitude of theirs.

So we pretended nothing was happening. Everyone around him did the same thing. That last period of his life was good. We've got videos of him ...

Mark You tried to go on as if nothing was happening?

Con Exactly. That was the way my wife and daughter wanted it. But on reflection, I was a mess. I just broke down, I just couldn't wear it.

The hardest thing I ever had to do was when my

wife and I and my daughter went in to tell him he had cancer, that was about two days after he'd been diagnosed, and we had to tell him that he had cancer.

He looked up and he said: 'But I couldn't have cancer, Dad, I'm too young. I'm too young to have cancer. I'm too young to die.'

I said: 'Don't worry, we'll give it everything we can. It's serious shit, mate, but it's not impossible.' But I knew in my heart it was. But we had to try. You always live in that hope that tomorrow someone's going to come out with a miraculous bloody cure for it. It's happened in the past. People with incurable diseases ...

There must have been a big group of people at the point of time when they come up with these cures, who were at the right place at the right time and were able to get it in time. You always live in that hope. So I figured the more we could keep him alive, however slim the chance of finding a cure for this shit, then we had a duty to try to do that, to him and ourselves. Well, to him mainly.

I handled it even worse than them in the sense that because I was the head of the family, and I had read all the stuff I could and I knew the realities of it, but I had to go along with it. The hardest thing was not telling him. I keep reproaching myself for not telling him, then I think I did the right thing by not telling him.

Mark What would you have gained if you had told him?

Con Nothing. Nothing. All we would have gained is that I reckon he would have given up the ghost and lasted two months instead of six or seven months.

Mark Do you think Sam had the time to realise he was dying and do the sort of things he wanted to do?

Con Yes. We gave him all the time. Whatever time he had, he did what he wanted to do. We were very lucky because of my position. I'm not exactly broke. We were able to go overseas. We were able to see things. We could have his friends over all the time. It's not as if he had a house, or money, or anything. He lived at home with us. So he had no affairs to put in order.

He graduated from grade 12 at Nudgee College there, and in late November or early December we went to Nudgee and got his certificates. We did all of that sort of stuff.

See this picture? That was his car. I bought it for him while he was sick. He thought it was just fantastic. He drove it twice.

Mark Tina, can you tell me about the start of it all?

Tina Sam had normal X-rays. We went to see the specialist who ended up operating on his spine, and he said Sam was overweight and had a bad back—that sort of thing. He told him he'd better lose weight or he might require surgery.

So Sam went on a diet, but he lost weight too fast. He lost about 10 kilos in four weeks, which is pretty fast considering that normally he'd found it difficult to lose weight.

But he didn't lose all that much weight at the end, just muscle really. He would still have been a big boy. He probably would have weighed about 90 kilos, maybe 98.

Con He would have been more than that.

Tina No, he was 110 kilos last time he was on his feet.

Con But he didn't waste away.

Tina No, but his muscle did.

Mark How tall was he?

Con About 6'2', maybe 6'3' [1.88–1.90 m].

Mark You said he grew quickly. How much?

Tina He would have shot up a foot in a year. Because every time I'd pick him up from Nudgee I'd think: 'God, he's getting tall!' He'd just keep growing and growing and growing.

Con He was boarding, you know. He was a hard-headed

little bloke, in the sense that he was a homebod. When
he was home he would just lie in front of the TV, muck
around, relax. He wouldn't study.

So we decided we'd send him to Nudgee College as
a weekly boarder. We'd pick him up Friday night after
school and take him back Sunday night. That's why,
apart from holidays, we wouldn't see him for the whole
week. So his mother would be able to see how much
he grew.

You ask the questions, because otherwise we'll just
ramble.

Mark   Part of the idea is to let you ramble, because you'll
tell me things I wouldn't have thought of asking.

The type of things I want people to talk about is how
they cope with the diagnosis of cancer. What did the
word cancer mean to you? Did it just mean he was sick?
Did it mean he was going to die? What did it mean to
you?

Con   It was a bit different for Tina than for me.
Because I'm the head of the household, I feel the
responsibility. I'm a lawyer and I deal in this sort of
stuff and I deal in injury cases. I know about
prognosis and that sort of stuff. When they told me
about the cancer I went and did a little bit of
reading, and I knew in my heart he was gone. I knew
there was really nothing we could do. I remember
coming home after the first couple of nights and we
just kept getting worse news.

nbFirst night they thought it might be lymphatic,
and they checked it. Then Dr Bill Parker, well, he
gave us a bit of hope, really. He said it might not be
Ewing's. Then the next day the results came through
and it was Ewing's. Then Dr Beadle was pretty well
straight with us from the word go. He more or less
said to me there was no hope.

I just came in and sat in this chair and bawled for
hours. I couldn't handle it. Tina came home and saw

me and got right up me. She called me a wimp and an arse and a donkey and all the rest of it. Then she said: 'We both know how serious it is, we know that. But while he's alive we're not going to grieve him.'

Tina Sam's attitude was always great, until he lost [the use of] his legs. He always had a great attitude. People sometimes say that cancer is caused by your attitude, but Sam's attitude to life was just brilliant. You couldn't have found a more easy-going relaxed person than Sam.

When I found out—when he had his first scan and nobody knew what it was, there was a radiologist who was pregnant, and of course they don't say anything, but she was watching the scan as she was taking the pictures. And I was watching her. And I was watching everybody around me, because mothers have got this ability to do that.

Nobody was saying anything, and as soon as I'd look at them they'd turn away. As soon as the picture of his knee came up on the screen, she sat down really heavily in a chair and let out a sigh. I thought: 'Hello, this isn't good.'

After that scan, the specialist said there was a growth there of some sort and it didn't look good. Because I know him, and he'd treated me in the past and I felt like I could talk to him pretty frankly, so I said to him: 'What is the worst scenario?' He said: 'Ewing's.'

I asked what it was and he explained it to me and I said: 'And what percentage chance do you give it of being that?' He said he wouldn't like to say because not all the tests had been done and so on. But I pressed him and he said: 'About 60 per cent.'

So then I knew. I knew from the word go what it was, and what hope he had.

But because of Sam's attitude, I put it at the back of my mind. We decided to go full speed ahead with whatever had to be done, and make it the happiest time possible.

Mark Sam wanted to keep trying and fighting the whole time?

Tina Oh, yes. The whole time. Because Sammy couldn't walk when they diagnosed him, but with chemotherapy he was getting better and he got to the stage where he was almost normal. He didn't want to handle it any other way. I don't think he wanted to dwell on the fact that it was going to be serious in the long run, although I do believe that he basically knew.

Con We never told him.

Tina But he did know. He used to talk to his friends about it. But he didn't want to dwell on the fact.

Con He just didn't want anyone else to worry about him. He was that sort of a kid.

Tina He didn't want anyone to visit him who he didn't normally see. You can imagine, being Italian, all the relations you haven't seen for ages want to come over and . . . you know. But Sam wouldn't have a bar of that, and I wouldn't either. They probably thought I was quite a bitch, but I wouldn't allow anybody near him unless they had as natural an attitude as possible.

Because that's what Sammy wanted. Even when he was flat on his back in bed, and he couldn't walk because of the pain, if anybody walked in who showed the wrong face—his grandfather or Con or anyone—he'd say: 'Mum, get rid of them. Just tell them to go away.'

That's basically how we handled it. Because we knew the seriousness of it, there was no time for mucking around, there was no time for emotional outbursts, there was none of that.

We just knuckled down, hoped for the best, hoped for a miracle, but in the meantime we all kept as positive an attitude and as happy an environment as we could.

Con   Tina and I broke down only once in front of him, didn't we?

Tina   Actually, we cried with him. He was upset because he realised that things weren't going well. I cried with Sam, but I never cried for him.

Mark   You said that at one stage he couldn't walk, then he got better. Did you think then that he was cured?

Tina   No, but we did think he was in remission. Even the doctor said that because he got well so fast, they thought that maybe they had contained the thing somehow. So we all thought we were containing it. And the second lot of scans said it hadn't spread very far.

In patches where there had been little ones, he didn't have them, but he had little ones in other areas. Basically it was being contained at one stage. We were hoping that this would continue.

Con   But then it just got worse and worse and worse.

Mark   Was it hard to stay positive when it must have been putting so much strain on your own relationship and your relationships with Zina?

Tina   Actually, we didn't seem to have too many problems like that, did we? I mean Con's work suffered, everybody's social life suffered, but it's totally irrelevant.

Con   Nothing else mattered.

Tina   But not only that, his friends were a big help. The thing that's very important for a patient like that is for their friends to be around. The people of their own age that they can identify with.

I know when Sammy was getting really sick, he went through a stage where he didn't want to see his friends. I sat down and had a talk to him and said: 'It would be much easier for your friends to stay away than it would be for them to come and see you. To them, you're the same old Sam, regardless of whether you can walk or whether you can talk or whatever. You put yourself in their position. If one of your best friends was sick, it would be easier to abstain from going to visit them. It would be easy for me to run away, too.

'But for them to come and want to stay with you, it's because they really do care about you. You should see it that way rather than the fact that in your eyes your body isn't functioning normally.'

He got over that, and allowed them to come and see him again. Throughout his whole illness they were always here. Always. Even if they weren't in the same room as him, they were always around. That was very important to him. I think that's what kept him in high spirits. They'd include him in their plans, and tell him what they were going to do, and they'd go out to dinner every night of the week when Dad wasn't here, when he could walk. They always planned different activities. They were as normal as possible—I think that helped.

Mark It seems sometimes brothers and sisters can feel neglected and forgotten. Did that happen?

Tina The thing with brothers and sisters at that age is that they never have a kind word to say to each other, but they love each other to death. But the language, well, it was rather coarse at timcs. They called each other some rather unsavoury things. But they stuck up for each other. Zina would cover for Sam, and Sam would cover for Zina if ever we were away and they wanted to go out with their friends without our permission. They were thick as thieves, but not demonstrably so.

When Sammy first got sick Zina left work and came home and stayed with me until Sammy was on his feet and normal again. Because Sam was telling us all to piss off and do our own thing. He'd say: 'Dad, get Zina out of here, tell her to go to work!'

Then they all went back to work, and everything was fine, but when Sammy started getting sick again Zina took time off work. She just couldn't concentrate on work knowing Sammy was sick at home. It was the best thing she could have done.

In a situation like that, it depends on the individual. But had Zina not taken that time off work and looked after her brother the way she did, I think she would have found it a lot more difficult to cope with when he left.

I don't think she's ever felt she could have done more.

Con That's the key. The key to trying to cope with this sort of thing is that you must feel satisfied in your own mind that at the end of the day, you've done everything possible.

Tina But some people aren't in a position where financially they can do everything they want. Luckily we didn't have that problem.

Mark Were there things that you think could have been done differently? Or that you should have done, but didn't?

Con I can't think of a single thing we could have done. And I don't know that we would have done it any different.

I think if we'd have told him: 'Sam, you've got cancer, it's terminal, you're going to die', then I think he would have gone a lot earlier, and it would have been against the way that he always felt. If we had given up on him straight away, it would have demoralised him.

I just can't see any other way that we could have done it, can you Tina?

Tina We were very lucky because I have a nephew who Sammy really looked up to. He's 23 and he lives down south and my son really looked up to him. Robert's a real scalliwag and he's very physical and always happy. Well, when Sammy was diagnosed Robert came up for four weeks to help us look after Sam. And when Sammy got on his feet again, then Robert went home.

Then when Sammy went downhill again, Robert turned up.

Con   He stayed with him until he died.

Tina   As soon as Sam knew Robert was coming, well, it was the first time we'd seen him smile in weeks. He lit up, and this mischievous look came in his eyes. We're very lucky that there were so many friends and family that we could include.

Con   In most cases, people wouldn't be able to cope. We kept him at home with us, but it took four or five people to move him from here to the bedroom next door. It was a major operation, because he was so big and heavy. You couldn't inflict too much pain on him, even though he was on morphine and Endone and God knows what. But we had the people available.

Even just a few days before he died, we took the whole lot outside. We could move him and . . . they get so uncomfortable that last couple of weeks. Nothing that you do makes them comfortable. In Sam's case, he could only feel his arms and up, nothing below that.

I think God looked after him in that sense. If he could feel his chest and back and legs for that last two months, when the pain really set in, I don't know how he would have coped. He would have had to have been knocked out to have coped with it.

Tina   Sammy was very tolerant of the pain, wasn't he? He never ever complained about anything.

Con   What Tina is saying is that we were fortunate in that we didn't have to put him away in a hospice and wait for him to die, because we didn't have the wherewithal to be able to look after him. We had the physical assistance. The Blue Nurses would come once or twice a day, but basically we did everything. Tina and I and Zina and Rob, we did everything.

Tina   He didn't let me out of his sight for a minute. He

had every gory test you can imagine, and we had to be there. There were times when I felt like running away and leaving him to it but, you know, he'd be saying to the doctors: 'My mother is staying.' He'd tell them all: 'My mother is staying.'

Con   We stayed with him. When he was in hospital we stayed with him. Tina and I would take turns. One night Tina would stay with him, another night I'd stay. They gave us a double room—we had this whole double room to ourselves. It was so good that we could stay there with him and help him the whole time.

Tina   I wouldn't leave Dr Beadle alone with Sam, because Dr Beadle was very concerned to see that Sam knew exactly what was going on. Geoff was just brilliant, he was very kind, but he was concerned that Sam didn't know what was going on. He wanted to give Sam the facts in black and white.

But from the beginning I said to him: 'You're not going to go in there cold turkey and tell our kid he's going to die.' We said to play it by ear according to his personality and how he was. We'd tell him, of course, but not tell him the brutal truth until the end. Geoff didn't agree with that.

At the initial interview Geoff said that he had to tell him. I said: 'Tell him, but don't say that there's no hope. You tell him that he's got cancer, and that it's going to be tough, fine, but don't tell him what the end result is going to be.' Because for an eighteen-year-old kid who hasn't done anything, it's very hard.

I don't know whether we were being ultraprotective or not. Knowing his personality, you just couldn't say something like that straight out to him.

Geoff said to us: 'You know, I'll eventually get the chance to talk to him on my own' and I said: 'Well I've got news for you—we're not leaving him for a second.'

Con   But they accepted that.

Tina   They thought it was wonderful. Because after he got

to know Sammy ... I said to him: 'You think I'm wrong, but make an effort to get to know Sammy. At the moment he's just another one of your patients. But after you've got to know him, then you can tell me whether I'm right or wrong.' And he did. He got to know Sam pretty well, and they'd joke and carry on.

I think he would probably agree now with the way we handled it, rather than break it to him like that.

Mark If he was 21 or 23 or 25 and still living here the same way, do you think you would have told him earlier? Did you keep it from him because of his age or his personality?

Tina I probably would have been more up-front ... I don't know. That's hard. That's a hard one.

Con He was a very young eighteen.

Mark At what stage would you have treated him as an adult? At what stage would you have told him what was going on, explained what he had to deal with, offered all the support possible, of course, but basically made it his responsibility to deal with?

Tina He would probably have never been an adult in my eyes.

Con Sam always relied very heavily on us.

Tina Sammy was a homebody. Zina and I were totally excited when, at the age of seventeen, he brought home a friend. Sam was a homebody. Sam would never stay at anybody's house. Sam would never have anybody stay here.

We used to worry about him. Why isn't he like normal kids who take off from home and do their own thing? But he was the total homebody.

Con Sam was a young eighteen. He was happy and comfortable with us taking control. He was still a kid.

Tina But he had the wisdom of a very old person, at times. As he grew up and got taller than me, I always saw him on a par to me. Mainly because he made me feel so petite, and I've never felt that way.

No, he was very smart, very cunning, but very laid back. He didn't worry about the things normal people worry about, yet he was a worrier. People getting physically hurt, or death, they used to worry him.

Con   A couple of weeks before he was diagnosed, the kid he sat next to at Nudgee College jumped off the Gateway Bridge and suicided. Then a while later another one did the same. And he said: 'You know Dad, it's funny. Here I am fighting for my life, and there's people throwing theirs away.'

Mark   I wanted to ask you something Con discussed before. In your mind, were you going to see the Pope because you really thought it would help, or because you thought you had to try everything you could.

Tina   I went there thinking we had to try everything we could. I didn't have any false expectations. I'm a lot more realistic than that. Mind you, I was hoping, too. But not to the degree where I really expected something.

Mark   But you're glad you went?

Tina   I'm glad that we did it the way we did. If it had been just the three of us or four of us, it probably would not have been as good mentally for Sammy. But we were lucky that two of his cousins came and his best friend and my daughter's best friend, so it was a whole heap of young kids travelling around. He enjoyed it. I'm glad that's the way we did it. That was the ultimate way to do it.

Mark   So it was a holiday with a couple of stopovers on the way.

Tina   Yes, with his friends. Always keeping that youth present. Kids he loved and trusted. The presence of those people was very important.

Con   There's a lot of books saying that you can beat cancer just by having a positive mind. We thought that letting him know we were going to find a cure in a spiritual sense, it was all part of a scenario of trying to keep him positive. In many respects, it was trying to keep us positive, too.

Apart from anything else, we just wanted to be together with him. I don't know what Tina feels, but I just felt good being with him.

I never even changed their nappies when they were babies. I'm not like you New Age blokes, I used to leave it all up to Tina. If the kids were crying when they were babies, it was: 'Tina, go and get them.' There was no way I'd ever pick them up.

Tina What are you talking about? If the kids were crying when they were adults it was: 'Tina go and get them.'

Con But if there was anything that made me love him so much, it was to do things for him. He'd say: 'Dad, Dad, Dad, I gotta hang a piss, Dad.' So you'd go and help him do a piss. And it would leak a bit and I'd say: 'Sorry, mate' and he'd say: 'Dad, you're bloody hopeless at this.' He'd say things to me like: 'Dad, I love you for what you're doing for me.'

Tina He was always telling us things like that. 'You're the greatest Mum and Dad in the world,' he'd say. Always. All the time. When we were trying to move him, he'd say: 'Don't. Stop. You'll do your back in. I'm killing my family.'

He wouldn't allow us to lift him or move him if he didn't feel we were doing it right. That's where Robert used to come in, because Robert was a young guy, pretty muscly. Sam would give us instructions. 'Let Robert do it.'

He was always good humoured, you know. Even to the very end.

Con Even the morning that he died, he was still trying to fight it. Even during that last day, when the morphine had got to him and he was nearly unconscious, he was still trying to fight it. He never stopped fighting it until the end.

But he went along with us all the way. He went along with everything that he thought would be a help. We put him on this paw paw juice for the last couple of weeks, and it was terrible!

Tina He drank the most revolting concoctions. If it was Zina, she would have thrown up. But Sammy would take the most revolting medicines without complaining.

Con But everybody was just marvellous. Like Geoff Beadle. Even at the end when we had the big foundation lunch* you know, he'd see so many patients, so many, and so many of them would die . . .

We took him out to dinner to say thank you and we especially invited him to come to this foundation lunch, and he's just not the sort of bloke to do that. He said to me: 'I don't do this.'

But he took an interest because, and Rosendahl [the GP] will tell you the same thing, that these people don't normally see the things that Tina and I and the family did for our son. Not because we're any better or because we're special, but because it's our culture to do it. He's part of us, and we've got to help him as much as we can. If there's such a thing as dying peacefully with as much support and love as you can get, then we were able to offer that to Sammy. He died in that room next to you.

But in terms of coping with it, I cope with it one way, Tina copes with it another way.

Tina Sam's attitude to life was this—as long as you're comfortable and happy, then just blunder through. And I think that's what we did—blundered through. Without trying to think about the horrible too much.

When I was home sometimes with Sammy I would look at him and try to imagine what it would be like

---

* The lunch raised money to start the Sam Sciacca Foundation.

with him not here. I thought I could get a fairly good idea.

But it's nothing like it. The reality of it is nothing like what I imagined. And I'm a fairly realistic sort of person.

The permanence of it—that's the horrible part. Initially you feel relieved because they're not suffering any more. You feel sadness, but you feel relieved just as much. But afterwards you have to realise it's permanent. You realise they're not coming back. I'm still realising that, actually. I still have to remind myself he won't be back.

Con It's not something you can really share. You can't share this pain. It's hard to share.

Tina But we knew Sam differently. He knew him as his father. I knew him not only as his mother, but also as a friend and as a person who he tried to shock on many occasions, and it didn't work. So he'd tried to shock me some more. I knew the sort of music he liked ... you know, things mothers know that fathers don't.

Even now when I get in his car sometimes and go and visit him, he plays me one of his favourite Midnight Oil or one of his favourite U2 numbers, or his favourite Police numbers. It's like he's telling me: 'Come on Mum, snap out of it, I'm still around.'

They're the little benefits that I've got that Con hasn't got, because Con wouldn't know those sorts of things. Most fathers don't, when they're busy and working. So one of the good things about being at home is that you learn all these things about your children that you wouldn't otherwise learn. And I was home with him all the time.

Con Whenever I'm home, I'll go and sit down with him at the cemetery, have a cigar with him. There's not a day that I'm home that we don't go and see him. That's how we're coping. It's not him, it's just bones. But you feel it's him. It's only been seven and a half months.

Tina I feel more comforted here at home than at the cemetery. I feel him more here. There's all these different things. I dream of him where Con doesn't.

Con I can't. I try really hard. But I just can't dream of him.

Tina There's lots of little things that you can't explain that happen that make you more content knowing that there is something there that you can't explain. On two occasions, Zina and I have had exactly the same dream about Sam. Exactly. The same night, the same dream. That's really strange. I still feel he's around.

And when we were in Greece that time I had a near death experience, and I wasn't dead. Those little things keep me comforted. It doesn't make up for the fact that he's not around, physically.

Mark Do you think your religion helps? Do you believe you're going to see him again?

Tina Yes. Regardless of whether I'm good or bad, I believe I'll see him again.

Mark Is that a comfort?

Tina I don't know ...

[Brad and Gavin, two of Sam's friends, arrived. Another friend, Simon, arrived later. They all visit regularly.]

Con Tina believes that. I believe the whole gambit.

Tina Con's religious beliefs are a little different to mine. Con is gung ho. To the book. To the letter. I was brought up in a Catholic school, so I have my own sceptical ideas.

Con I just don't believe there was any other reason, though. You can't be sceptical, because if you start looking at it all in a logical sense then you might as well not believe in anything. Religion has no logic. You can't really be logical if you believe in religion. There are a few logical parts, but if you believe in heaven, hell, the resurrection, life after death and all that, then it really is a faith. Because there's nothing logical or scientific to say it's true—in fact, science would say the opposite.

But if you can't believe in that, if you can't have faith in that, then there doesn't seem to be any sense or purpose in life. If you're just here then you go, then you're gone. That's it.

But I believe that every one of us has a different character, a different being, a different way we operate, and I don't believe that can die. It's your spirit, although not in a religious sense. I can't believe physical things make you what you are. They may make you walk and talk and do all those things mechanically, but it can't make what you are.

The Christian Church has been around for 2000 years. Empires have gone down the tube in a couple of hundred years, so there must be something there. If you read a lot of this stuff, and you do see the documented miracles where there's no explanation for what happened, then it's good for you to believe in it. And you can think to yourself: 'Shit, he's not gone. If I lead a fair life, I'll see him again'.

That's where Tina and I differ. I think if I'm bad, I'm not going to see Sam. It's as simple as that.

Tina   I don't think that happens.

Mark   Can you see a purpose in him dying? Can you say that this is God's plan?

Tina   No. I'm very angry about that. Con can, but I can't. I can't find any reasons to justify him not being here. I'll never forgive God for that. It's something I just won't forgive him for.

Con   Well, God doesn't need you to forgive him. The point is that if there is such as thing as God, and I believe that there is, well you still say to yourself: 'Why? Why would anyone want to take him away?'

I don't agree with it, and I'd much rather he was here. But seeing as though he's gone, it's better for me to be able to believe. It makes me feel better to believe there had to be a plan here.

Mark Even if you know that you're rationalising, it still helps?

Con Yes. What's the point of being angry for the rest of your life. You feel shithouse about it, and you say: 'Why did you do it here?', but at the same time you think that there may have been a reason for it. I don't know what it is, and I can't understand it, and I don't agree with it, and I'm angry too, but at the end of the day that sense of anger is not going to bring him back. So to try to get some peace, you try to rationalise it. I don't like it, but at least there may have been a reason. That's all part of having faith.

I prefer to believe that to being angry, or to believe nothing. Of course I'm angry, and of course if I could change it I would change it. If I had the choice I'd say I want him here. I don't want him somewhere bloody else.

Anne-Louise Van Den Nieuwenhof

Interview with Anne-Louise Van Den Nieuwenhof, aged eight, and her parents Christine and Ray in their Sydney home. Also present were Tim six, Mary-Ellen five and Michael three months.

Christine Anne-Louise turned five in February, and a month after her fifth birthday she was diagnosed with a Ewing's tumour. Her fifth birthday was uneventful, we had our usual picnic in the park with family and friends, and she was just starting school, then but about a week after that she started complaining of shoulder pain. One day it was sore, then it wasn't, then I'd dry her at night after a shower or bath and then it would be sore, then it wasn't. In the meantime she was still climbing trees and swinging off the clothesline.

Then she woke up two nights in a row with this shoulder pain and I gave her some Panadol, but it didn't help. So I took her to the local doctor and he ordered some X-rays. Coming out of the X-ray office, being the trained nurse, I just thought I'd have a look at the report and see what it said. The X-ray showed either a Ewing's, a histiocytoma, an osteogenic sarcoma or osteomyelitis. Well I knew she didn't have osteomyelitis because she didn't have a temperature and she didn't seem all that sick, so I thought it had to be either the Ewing's or the osteogenic sarcoma or the other one.

We went down to our local doctor—he'd already been contacted by the results department and he knew what they were. He referred us to Michael Stevens at the Children's Hospital. We went down next day, and saw him, and about a week after that she started chemotherapy. She was treated with local radiotherapy for five weeks and chemotherapy for two years. They talked about surgery—amputation to try to control the tumour in her arm—but when she was re-assessed at the end of the radiotherapy the tumour had shrunk and the chances of her needing amputation were smaller. At each re-staging she was just showing improvement.

So that's the technical events leading up to it all.

Mark   What was your initial reaction to the news?

Christine   Initial shock. I got home and I was very matter of fact. I thought I must let everyone know what this terrible X-ray showed up. So I rang my mother and told her, and she came down, and I rang Ray's parents, and they came over. It wasn't really disbelief, I mean we knew that those X-rays had to be real. We went off to the oncology unit next day knowing our child had some form of cancer.

I think the biggest shock was not reading the report

but walking into the oncology day clinic. We were waiting in the waiting room and there were about a dozen children without hair, looking quite pale. But they were normal, and they were playing, and they were climbing over the seats and they were eating. They weren't sick, well, they looked bloody sick, but they were just normal children sitting around drawing. And the parents were coping quite well, they were just sitting around chatting, and I thought maybe it won't be so bad after all.

Mark You said that was a shock. What did you expect?

Christine I expected it all to be, well, it was pretty horrific, but I expected it to be much worse. While she was going through her treatment I thought she'd be much sicker than she was. Somehow I thought the children would all be in wheelchairs, and not running around looking as well as they did. They were all coping so well, that really surprised me.

That was the reality of it. Here we were, we were one of these people that this never happens to, and here were we with these other twenty parents, trying to be really brave for Anne-Louise's sake. It wasn't until we saw Michael Stevens, and I had my sunglasses on, and he said: 'Do you mind taking your sunglasses off?', and I said: 'No, I like my sunglasses'. I felt really secure with my sunglasses on because underneath I'd been crying and my eyes were really red.

He said: 'This is not the first time I've been with someone whose child has got cancer. You *can* take your glasses off and you *can* cry, and don't try too hard to put on a front for Anne-Louise. It's good for her to know you're upset.' So with that I thought she was going to be faced with the truth sooner or later, so we might as well start being honest with her right now. So that's what we were.

We told her what was wrong with her, and all along we kept her informed of what was happening.

It was still her disease, and she had to look after it. Honesty was really important. And for the other children, we decided life had to be normal, or as normal as possible. Looking back on it, how on earth it could ever have been normal, I don't know. But we always had our evening meal together, whether it was here at home or down at the hospital, and whether Anne-Louise could be with us or not.

I think we expected too much from Anne-Louise. For the first week she was in and out, staying overnight sometimes. And even when her chemo started, we came home overnight. Being a children's nurse, but out of that sort of nursing for years, it was never policy for parents to stay overnight. That was never allowed.

So we used to stay until 11 o'clock when she settled down, then we'd go home. We told her we were only twenty minutes away, and the nurse would ring us if you need us, and we'd be back first thing in the morning. This went on for about two weeks. Poor child, when I think of her sitting in bed, having her chemo, and here was Mum and Dad at 11 o'clock packing up their bags and going home. It wasn't until we were about three weeks into our treatment that the doctor said: 'I believe you're not staying overnight.' And we said: 'Our child's quite used to it, she's independent, she can cope on her own, she's mature enough to know that we will be back.'

But it wasn't until then that we realised things were much more serious and her needs were much greater as a sick child than they were as a normal child.

Ray   When I walked into Wade House one morning, I was confronted by Dr Stevens, who was just about to get into the lift. He said 'Come and sit down here, I want to talk to you.' He said: 'Do you realise it's hospital policy for one of the parents to sleep with their child overnight?' He was telling me the policy after the event. He said: 'From now on, we expect one of you to stay in hospital with her while she's having treatment.' That was quite a shock because here's this doctor who's given us all the bad news about Anne-Louise having cancer, he's the one that's treating her and he's the one who's involved in it all, then he just pulls the rug out from under my feet. I felt really bad after that because I had put all this trust in him, and I had him up there in my estimation, and all of a sudden he's correcting our behaviour.

Christine But then as a mother, I really should have thought more about it. How can you expect your child to have cancer and be sitting up in a hospital bed on her own without us around. Anne-Louise, did you feel lonely?

Anne-Louise Yes.

Christine But you didn't tell us you felt lonely?

Anne-Louise No.

Mark Did you feel the staff had certain expectations of you as a parent?

Christine Oh, yes. But I felt as though I could do what I want, and I didn't feel scrutinised, and wouldn't have cared what they thought about me anyway. In a lot of ways they left us alone. The nurses there gave the medication but otherwise they relied on me to keep an eye on her.

Mark Did you get much help with people explaining what was going on?

Christine No. We had our own patient record—we held Anne-Louise's record and that had a list of the treatment she had and we carried that with us and we knew what was going to happen next week and six weeks down the line—but as far as knowing more about Ewing's, we've found that everything we've ever been to they've talked about leukaemia or solid tumours, but it's never been specific for Ewing's tumour.

But around that time in one of the hospitals I went to there was a medical journal lying around and in there was actually an article on Ewing's sarcoma. I've still got that. I mean, that was just a dream. Through Anne-Louise's whole treatment, that was my reference. I really clung to that, because that was the only thing that was just about Ewing's. We didn't know anyone with Ewing's, apart from this man that we met down at Ulladulla. Actually the fourth child she shared with had a Ewing's tumour, but he had a relapse and a bone marrow transplant and he died. That was pretty scary, too.

When we asked for the results of tests, they would give them to us. And when we asked for the results of other treatments, they would say it was difficult because there really wasn't enough Ewing's around to know and to perform the proper studies in Australia. They had to rely on what they could learn from overseas. This article that I read, actually, was written by an American doctor.

During treatment, well, it went much better than we expected. There were about six weeks of trying to get into the swing of things, then it's easier because you know what to expect, you know the results of the first induction chemotherapy. We knew what to expect each time after that. By the next round of chemotherapy we'd almost become blase, knowing what to expect and what reactions she could get. She used to have a three-week period of nothing before she'd start the next lot of chemotherapy and I never liked that time because it meant we weren't fighting anything. Couldn't we get on with it?

I always looked forward to the next round of chemo because it meant we were getting closer to fighting these creepy-crawlies that were crawling around. I used to almost look forward to getting on with our treatment. She had a five week cycle, then three weeks off, then five weeks back on, and so on.

Mark Obviously at the start you would have been scared Anne-Louise was going to die. When did that feeling change?

Christine The loss of our eldest child . . . the thought of that was horrific, just horrific. The first two weeks I spent crying, not so much around the children but probably more on my own because the two little ones were at kindy—Mary-Ellen was only thirteen or fourteen months old. I was never emotional in at the hospital, but at home I was.

Ray It brought a lot of things back, too, because you had been diagnosed with cancer yourself. That was a horrific time for me, too, because at that stage I thought she was going to die, too. We'd been surrounded by cancer. In four years, there were four cases of cancer. There was Christine's Dad, and that hit her because they were very close, then there was Christine herself, shortly after that was Anne-Louise, and then soon after that there was my sister—she had cancer and had a breast removed. So we had four people, very close to us, all diagnosed with it. I coped with it by keeping a diary of what was happening. I wrote in it every night or put something in it, and I never stopped writing. That was how I coped with it all.

Mark Did you find that by putting your emotions in the diary, you did not have to deal with them as much during the day?

Ray A lot of the time, I could save up what I was feeling. That was how I coped with it. I wrote down the very first treatment she had, the very first vomit she had, I documented it all.

Christine The hair loss was something we were really dreading. How were we going to cope with that? We had told Anne-Louise what was going to happen, and she was in hospital when her hair fell out. When we arrived one day she had this huge plastic bag, and she was just pulling out her hair and putting it in there. But it just wasn't an issue. At the time the issue was that she had no white cells, and we were more concerned about that, than we were about the hair loss.

Mark   Anne-Louise, did it worry you losing your hair?

Anne-Louise   No ... well. I can't remember all that much. I remember pulling out my hair and putting it in my bag.

Ray   Her grandfather started to cry—he couldn't handle it. I remember that very very distinctly. He took it much harder than she did—she treated it as part of a joke— look! my hair's falling out.

Christine   She decided to pull it all out down the sides and leave a strip down the middle, but it only took three days for it all to fall out. It became a bit of a game— 'what part will I pull out next'. The reality of the severity of the illness didn't sink in for a lot of our friends and family until the hair loss. That's when they could see for themselves that it was serious. Anne-Louise, how were the kids at school?

Anne-Louise   Some of the first class kids used to call out to me 'Baldy, baldy' when I first went back to school. But I didn't really take any notice.

Christine   Honestly, I really don't think the hair loss was an issue for Anne-Louise.

Ray   There was the realisation that she had the cancer, but as long as she had her hair, she was just being treated for it. But it didn't really hit people what was going on until she started losing her hair. Then they really understood.

Christine   But I really think that for Anne-Louise, it was not a major problem.

Ray   No, not a major problem.

Christine   She didn't have hair for three years. She was

absolutely bald. Not a hair on her body. She wore a ribbon a lot of the time—in fact, she started off a trend. I don't think it was to distinguish male from female, I just think it was a part of body costuming that made her look nice. I don't think she was frightened people would think she was a boy. In the first year she'd often wear just jeans and a tracksuit top, and at school they just wore a navy tracksuit. It wasn't that she was worried about her gender—she just wore the ribbon as a fashion accessory.

But on the whole the kids at school were very good. The school was very supportive.

Ray   The reason was that Kim came over. Kim works at the Children's Hospital. What she does is . . .

Christine   She went around and spoke to the kids at her school and told them what was wrong with Anne-Louise, and then spoke to her class while she was in hospital, and they had some books that we donated to the library and the teacher read them. Her teacher was very aware of childhood disabilities and she treated Anne-Louise just like she was any other child. She was never taken out of anything and she was still expected to do sport, and to do her homework. We used to take work into the hospital for her.

Ray   So even though she missed a lot of school, she missed 55 days, she kept up. And the fact that Kim came around meant that when Anne-Louise went back to school, it wasn't as bad as it could have been. I mean, kids are kids, but it could have been worse.

Christine   I think a lot of the kids took on Anne-Louise as their responsibility, so if anybody said: 'You look funny without your hair', they'd be bashed up.

Ray   And they were good in the way that if she was really nauseous she could pop home for an hour or so, or if she was really tired they'd ring up and let me know and she'd come home for a sleep, because the school's just over the road.

Christine   There were quite a few older kids who thought: 'Poor little kindergarten child, she's got no hair and she's got cancer'.

Anne-Louise   Some kids would come over at little lunch and see that I was all right.

Mark   At one stage your main thought was 'she's going to die'. At some stage that changes to 'she's going to live'. When did that happen?

Christine   It was probably a year or so into treatment that I felt secure at all. After a year, I could see my child actually finishing her first three years at school. but it wasn't until her treatment had finished—and she's been off treatment now for eighteen months—for a while, say three or six months ago, that I could see her having her twenty-first birthday. I can see her travelling. I've told her not to get married until after she's thirty. I can actually see a future. But I can honestly say that's only in the last six months.

Mark   So you're thinking now in terms of a cure, rather than a treatment?

Christine   Yes, yes. During treatment we were just going for three months at a time. We'd have a scan every three months and we'd think 'well, we've got over that hurdle'. That's when I'd start looking forward to it and getting on with our next three months.

Those scans are terrible. You sit there and you look at the screen while she's having the scan and you get terribly picky about what you're seeing. You think 'My God, was that spot there last time?' Of course you don't have a clue what you're looking at.

At six months we started to think a little better, but it wasn't until a year or fifteen months after treatment finished that we could really start thinking normally about it all.

Everything's back to normal now. It's been normal for a year. We've got a baby brother and things are going to stay normal and they're not going to get bad again.

Ray As the old saying goes, if one member of the family has cancer, we all have cancer. We've all lived with it for a while. And they've told us that if it came back, there'd be nothing they could do for it. It's not good to get it in the shoulder because you can't operate because it's too close to the lungs. I mean, if you get it in the leg you can take the leg off.

Mark Are you still worried it's going to come back?

Anne-Louise I don't really worry because the doctors told me that if I get to next year, I'll be all right.

Christine Anne-Louise knows that she's got until March next year, then her two years off treatment are up. She was told that.

Another thing that was important was to keep life as normal as possible for these other two. I was paranoid about the whole family being in turmoil because Anne-Louise was sick. It was really a priority to not protect them, but to continue on and let them know that they weren't going to be in turmoil. We were so busy for the first year having a really good quality life.

We used to come home from the hospital and we'd go for a picnic in the park, or we'd go to a restaurant for dinner, or we'd go feed the ducks. There was hardly a day, when Anne-Louise was well enough, that we weren't doing something. We'd go on bushwalks, or to friends' places to play. We had a great family life at the time, even though she was sick. But the time was so precious that we always thought we'd get in another picnic before she went for that treatment, or another bike ride.

Mark Do you think that helped?

Christine Yes, definitely. For Anne-Louise, the whole treatment became more positive. And you had to do things like that because often you'd go down to the hospital at 9 o'clock and you wouldn't start treatment or see a doctor until 3 o'clock. In that time, it was important Anne-Louise was kept busy. It wasn't trying to escape reality, but we would never just sit there and say we were sick of waiting.

We'd go for a walk to the university, or to the local pet shop, or the cake shop, or look at the nice houses and gardens. And we'd read and read and read. We'd play games. It was really important the whole treatment was positive and we were attuned to the positive feelings, rather than the negative side of it. That kept us going.

Mark   You made the effort to keep all the kids together?

Christine   Yes, often we'd have our family meals down at the hospital. That was really important. If we couldn't have it at home, we'd have it down there. A lot of the time we'd take Anne-Louise to the parents' dining room with us. If we couldn't, we'd go back to her bedside and have her evening story beside her bed and then the two little ones would come home with me and Ray would stay the night, or the other way around.

But it's always been *her* disease, not mine or Ray's. When we'd go to the clinic I'd tell Anne-Louise she had to answer the questions, or I'd drop her off at scanning and she'd let them know she was there. She's at the stage now where it's her disease, and she has to cope with it and know what's going on.

She knows that her chances of having children are diminished because she's had chemotherapy, and her chances of getting a second cancer are increased. We'd like to think she's aware—because we've always been very open—of the effects on fertility and growth and so on.

She's always been treated as a normal child. We have never made an allowance for her because she had cancer. She's always gone to school—she might have woken up saying she didn't feel well but I made her go to school and said that if she wasn't well in an hour she could come home.

But she was always happy to go school, which is something to do with the innocence and naivety of a five year old. Nothing will keep them away from school. Although some days she'd be back at lunchtime with a vomit bowl tucked under her arm. But she'd have a rest for an hour then go back.

Mark   What sort of reaction did you get from your family and friends? Did anybody turn away?

Christine   I had a few reactions like that from school. A lot of the ethnic people would come up and talk to me as if she had worms and their children would catch it if they played with her. One woman came up and told me her child had nits and she was sure she'd caught it from Anne-Louise.

Our families were very supportive. Ray's parents were very supportive—they used to share the duties of going down and looking after her. My family was supportive. I had a few friends who denied it, who didn't want to talk about it. Even now they say 'what a brave little girl', and that's the end of it.

Both our families are Catholics—I don't go to Mass, although Anne-Louise does sometimes, but we got a lot of religious things—we had prayers said for us, we had crosses, we had photos and relics, we had everything sent to us. So I put them all in this plastic bag and rather than the poor child wear all these things we used to put them under her pillow when she was in hospital or stick them behind her bed. There were photos of Mother Teresa, there was the Pope, Mother Mary McKillop, you name it. There were just heaps and heaps of these religious artefacts.

I didn't get anything out of my religion. It didn't come into it. I didn't pray for a cure. There was nothing there for me. Ray got a lot out of Petrea King.

Ray   Yes, Petrea King and that fellow in Melbourne, Ian

Gawler. Petrea King is in cancer support and I read all her books. I was on night shift and was able to do quite a bit of reading.

Christine Another fellow we went to was a naturopath/ herbalist. At no stage would we ignore the medical side, but we thought maybe a holistic approach could help, too. I don't know why we went.

Ray We were grasping for straws. I wrote to the Cancer Council and got every bit of information we could get. But at the time I was going through a bit of turmoil, coming home, not knowing who was going to get cancer next. I mean, four X-rays from the same X-ray place in Burwood, and four times it had been the locum because our doctor was away. I thought shit, what's next? Who's next?

Christine So next time we went for the holistic approach was when she had finished her treatment, we went off to a naturopath. I don't know why we went there—we wanted some safeguard because she was off treatment. In the end, she was only on his potions and lotions for six weeks, because she hated them. She said 'Now that I've finished treatment, why are you taking me to this fellow? Why am I taking these revolting medicines?' I think I was treating myself, rather than Anne-Louise.

Mark Did Anne-Louise struggle against the treatment, or did she accept it?

Christine For the first two years she went along fine but at the last five-week cycle she dug her heels in. We'd be driving down and she'd say: 'Why am I having this? I don't need this? Why do I have to go?' It was the last treatment, and she was really fed up. Probably through the last three months, but particularly in the last five weeks. She was beginning to hate it.

I never had to physically force her, and we never had to coax her. We'd just say: 'This is your last one, you know why we're doing this. If we get through this, then we're close to the end.' A few times she did refuse to have dexamethasone, which gave her an itchy bottom. She absolutely hated it. She would go into the clinic and the first thing she would say to the nurse was: 'I don't want the dexamethasone.'

And she had one psychotic attack, either from the dexamethasone or the largactil. She was trying to pull the drips out and get home. She was absolutely uncontrollable. But she doesn't remember it—when it was over she just lay down and went back to sleep.

The chemo she didn't mind—I think she'd rather vomit than have the dexamethasone and the itchy bottom. She never minded vomiting. She used to think that as long as she was vomiting, then the drugs were working and she would get better.

Mark   Was her illness a financial strain?

Christine   It was at first. Ray was working as a TNT security officer, doing shiftwork. That was ideal, because sometimes Ray was available in the morning, and sometimes in the evening, and I could juggle it around.

In the meantime, he'd applied for a job with Telecom and that came through. But you did have a bit of time off work, didn't you? And Ray couldn't work overtime.

I worked two nights a week and I probably missed two nights all up because of Anne-Louise being sick. But it was so important to go because going to work was so normal for me. I was there with my colleagues and my friends, and I made sure I kept that up. I think also when I look back on it, that going to work meant I was looking good. It meant I was coping with this kid with cancer, the kids were going to kindy and they were all right, my house was tidy, I could still go to work, nothing had changed, I was still strong, I could cope and I wanted to stay like that.

Mark   That's what you looked like, but did you feel like that inside or was that a bit of a show?

Christine   No, I probably didn't feel like that inside. I was thinking: 'God I hope this kid pulls through, I hope she's all right'. I was trying to keep life normal, but it was a cover-up.

Ray   It was all very hard on Tim. He was probably the most affected, even more than Anne-Louise. He developed a stutter.

Christine   The two little ones were devastated, because they'd always been together. They always wanted to know why we were going to the hospital, and what was happening to her—the whole conversation was why, when, why, when, what.

Ray   When she'd come home they'd all grab an ice-cream bowl each, so the three of them all walked around with vomit containers. And they'd rub her back when she was being sick, and if she vomited they'd want to vomit, too. They were all affected—it wasn't just Anne-Louise.

Christine   They were very good at the hospital. They'd come in and just sit with her quietly. We did a lot of good things in hospital. There were a lot of positive things to come out of it. As I said, we utilised every well moment. We read some great books, we played lots of nice games, the hospital had a recreationalist who came around and played with us. And we used to go on great holidays.

Ray   One of the first holidays we went on was down to Milton-Ulladulla—they've got a cancer house there. This was sponsored by Helen Bates, and I think Rotary had something to do with it. She takes a lot of first-time cancer kids. Last time we were down there 119 children with cancer had gone through. She's got a register of all the kids who have been there. It's the first chance parents get to be with their child after diagnosis. They encourage the families to get together for a holiday. She does a great job—just recently she was awarded an MBE for all her work.

Coming into contact with people like that was great,

and with Camp Quality as well, and all the people associated with that, and the Terry Fox run ...

Christine Even with all that, we got most of our support off each other. I went to work, and that helped me a lot, and Anne-Louise herself coped so well. Because she wasn't in hospital for long periods at a time, life was fairly normal for her apart from the times of chemo and then being sick for a few days after that. She was still going to school, and playing with her friends, and that kept us going. I had visions of having my child in the beanbag in the classroom, or having the teacher come over and give her lessons for an hour after school, but it wasn't like that. Physically she kept really well, and in some ways life went on perfectly normally. She never complained.

The only problem she had was the bath. She'd take her medicine, and have her drops, and have the chemo, but when she was supposed to have a bath she'd be kicking and screaming and uncontrollable. I felt like getting a hose and hosing you down.

Anne-Louise I hated the drip, too. I hated that.

Christine What do you think was the worst about it all?

Ray Yes, we've done enough talking. Let's hear it from you, Anne-Louise.

Christine She had a central line put in, and when the chemo went in it had been in the fridge, so it was cold. She used to hate the sensation of it travelling around the tube. Would that have been the worst?

Anne-Louise The butterflies were OK, but the fingerpricks hurt. I didn't like them.

Christine That's awful, watching your kids have a fingerprick, watching your child have all this barbaric treatment.

Mark Anne-Louise, were you scared about what was going to happen or were you just thinking about what was happening each day?

Anne-Louise I was thinking about what's happening now.

Mark You didn't worry about what was going to happen next week or next month or next year?

Anne-Louise No.

Mark So they were all the bad things, were there any good things?

Anne-Louise Well ... [long pause]

Ray There was a girl that did all the artworks who you liked.

Christine And all the friends you met.

Anne-Louise Yeah, friends. But the bad thing was I didn't go to school.

Ray She loved to learn.

Christine But then you got in contact with Camp Quality, which was good, and you went to Mollymook, which you enjoyed.

Anne-Louise Yes. I went on lots of holidays. And I liked the people at the Children's Hospital, and I went to the Gold Coast.

Christine I used to get worried for the other two when Anne-Louise went on all these fantastic trips. So I'd often take them to Mollymook for a fun-packed holiday and have a really good time with them. I felt really sorry for the other two when Anne-Louise went away, I really felt they were missing out.

But there were heaps of positive things that came out of it. She was on 'GP'—well, she was in the filming of it, anyway. They had a show on 'GP' about Camp Quality.

Anne-Louise I was really looking forward to it but I was only on for about two seconds. You only saw my shoes.

Christine For myself, there was a lot of things came out of it. We had a really valued two years. I enjoyed being with my child while she was sick, I met some nice people through there.

At one stage I went to the funeral of a 22-month-old girl who had leukaemia, and I thought: 'If I can handle this, I can handle anything.' It was the saddest affair I had ever ever been to. Things like that bring back the reality of it all. It's a real jolt. You realise that your kid was in the same boat at that time.

I found that really hard. A few times Anne-Louise has wanted to go to the funerals of different ones we've known, and I think she could cope with it, but I don't think I could cope yet.

We spoke about death when we needed to, but we didn't talk about it all the time. Occasionally Anne-Louise would say: 'Am I that sick I'm going to die?' and we'd say: 'No, you've got a long way to go before you're that sick.' And she never was that sick. She was never in intensive care or anything.

But we let her know when she was first diagnosed that could have happened; that if she didn't have treatment that could happen. We talked about death quite openly. We had lots of animals at the time and when the animals died they went to heaven and the kids would help bury them. We'd write notes to send up to all the dead people that we knew, and if we buried a chook the chook would have a stack of letters with it. At first that was a big part of our conversation. I was paranoid—I made sure she knew it was OK to die and it was OK to cry and there was nothing to be scared of and it was worse for the people left behind.

Mark Who made the decisions about treatment?

Ray When you're five years old, you can't make decisions like that. But she's older now, and it's different. She's already told us that if the cancer comes back, she won't have any more treatment. She's already told us that.

Mark Why is that, Anne-Louise?

Anne-Louise I saw someone in hospital who'd gone back for more treatment, and she had all these machines connected up to her and I thought: 'Oh no, is that what would happen to me?' I wonder if I'm going to die like that. I don't want to have all those machines around me. If you have all those machines, you still die. I'd rather die without those machines.

Christine   You'd rather die at home just like you are now, rather than hooked up to machines?

Anne-Louise   Yes.

Mark   Was there ever a time Anne-Louise was so sick you thought you should stop the treatment?

Christine   No, never.

Mark   You always thought it would work?

Christine   Yes, I had every faith in the doctors and whatever they wanted to do, they could go ahead and do it. I always questioned them about what they were doing and what the side effects were—I always wanted to know more. I asked them to give me as much information as they could.

Mark   Has it changed you?

Ray   I'm sure it's affected me. Things were just chaos with Chris getting cancer and having her operation just before Anne-Louise was diagnosed, having a new baby and having to express milk and mix it with formula to feed Mary-Ellen so Chris wouldn't get mastitis. It was just chaos. It's affected me, for sure. I've lost my memory, for one thing. It was chaos.

Christine   Things never get back to normal, really. I don't think they do. At night you go to bed and thank God we're all still here.

Ray   You learn to take one day at a time. Things that were important before are unimportant—that's one thing I've learnt. Take things as they are, and in their proper perspective.

You learn to value your health—you value the fact that you wake up and you're alive.

Mark   So do you feel like it's all over now, Anne-Louise?

Anne-Louise   Yes.

Mark   When did you start to think it was all over?

Anne-Louise   Well . . .

Christine   The statement of all statements came a couple

of weeks ago. Anne-Louise was getting ready to go to Camp Quality and Mary-Ellen was sitting there and she said: 'Oh Anne-Louise, I can't wait to get old and lose my hair so I can go to Camp Quality, too.'

Corinne Woollard

Interview with Corinne Woollard, aged 19, her parents Chris and Rod and her younger sister Pauline in their home on the south coast of NSW.

Corinne In October 1988 I found a lump at the top of my femur. It was growing pretty quickly so I went to the local doctor. They started tests, and I went to different doctors, and I had a biopsy and it was cancer. Then they started twelve weeks of chemo, then I had a bone replacement at the beginning of 1989. In 1991 the pin broke and they did a bone graft. That's basically it.

Mark So you didn't have any pain, just a swelling?

Corinne That's right. It grew from nothing to about the size of the palm of my hand in a few weeks. My school skirt just got tighter and tighter in a matter of weeks— that's how quickly it grew.

Mark What did you think was going on at the time?

Corinne I don't think I was worried about anything. I started to worry it might be cancer when I had the bone scan. That's when I found out—that's when Mum told me it was pretty sure to be cancer. The doctor had told her.

Rod Actually, you went to the chiropractor first. Remember?

Chris Yes, we thought it was something muscular.

Rod Then when that didn't do any good it was to the doctor, then for X-rays and bone scans. Once it was verified we saw the specialist in Wollongong on a

Friday, and on the Monday she was up [to Sydney] to
see Dr Marsden.

Mark So how long did it take from the time you first saw
a doctor to the time you started chemo?

Corinne A couple of weeks. It was pretty quick.

Mark And what did it mean to you when you were told
you had cancer. What did you think?

Corinne I don't think I was that worried about it. When I
was down getting the bone scan, that's when Mum told
me. It was just before I went in the room, so when I
went in I was all alone. There was nobody around, just
the machine ... But after that, it didn't really concern
me that much. I didn't think that much about it. I
don't think I really knew what was going on.

Mark So you thought: this is a minor problem, the
doctors will fix it.

Corinne Yep.

Mark How about you two?

Chris I don't think we were all that worried about it,
either. I don't think we were aware of the seriousness
of what type of tumour it was. We knew there was a
tumour there, but we thought it was just a matter of
getting some treatment and that would be it.

Rod Thinking about it, it's just as well we didn't have a
book. If I really knew what was going on, I think I'd
have cracked up a bit.

Mark Did it occur to you at any stage that it might have
spread somewhere else?

Chris No.

Rod Never. To me, the seriousness of it first dawned
when we went to Marsden, and he said the first priority
was to save her life, and the second priority was to save
her leg. How serious the cancer was hadn't dawned on
us until then. Then I was concerned.

Mark How about you, Pauline?

Pauline I didn't think about it the whole way through. I
was fourteen at the time, and I don't think I really

understood anything much. I knew she went to the doctors, and I knew she had to have all this treatment and it made her hair fall out, but it really didn't mean all that much.

Chris In some ways I was the only one that ever really saw her sick. I'd take her to Sydney for the chemo and she'd stay overnight, and she might be quite sick there. But by the time she got home and the others saw her she was starting to pick up and feel and look a bit better.

Mark So you had twelve weeks of chemo, then you had the operation. What did you have done?

Corinne They took out about 8 centimetres of bone and replaced it with ceramic discs and a Huckstepp pin.

Mark How long did it take you to start walking?

Corinne I was walking within a week, but I was on crutches for quite a while—about two months.

Mark Then did you have more chemo after that?

Corinne No, that was it. It was over pretty quickly.

Chris Because it hadn't spread anywhere, they didn't have to do anything more.

Corinne When I had that operation, they did some more tests and told me they couldn't find any trace of it. They didn't need to do radiation therapy.

Mark Were you told you were cured?

Corinne Once I had the operation and they told me there was no more cancer, I thought 'Fine'. I didn't expect there to be any more, anyway. I've had no problems— it didn't worry me much at all. It was one of those things—I didn't know what to expect so I took it as it came.

Mark So you never really worried that it would come back?

Corinne No.

Mark Chris?

Chris We think about it. We wonder a bit whether there will be a recurrence, but I wouldn't say we actually worry. I think I have to add that we're a Christian family and our belief that God is in control of our lives has made a big difference. If we hadn't had that faith, then I think it would have turned our lives upside down. Because even though we can't say this has happened for a particular reason, we know that God does bring things into our lives for particular reasons, and that has made a big difference to our acceptance of it.

Mark So would that have helped you accept things if the cancer hadn't been controlled?

Chris Yes. It still would have been devastating to us, but there would have been this reassurance that God was controlling things and that it was for a purpose, even if we couldn't see what it was.

Mark Corinne, what was the hardest thing about the whole episode?

Corinne Probably the needles. I was more worried each time about going and having the needles. I had a Portacath, where they put the needle in for the chemotherapy. Losing my hair didn't worry me too much at first, but later on it did a bit.

Mark Were you perfectly bald?

Corinne Yes.

Mark How long were you bald for?

Corinne It started growing back when I had the operation, so that was a couple of months.

Mark Was it the same when it grew back? You didn't have tight black curls? [Corinne has thick straight brown hair.]

Rod It's grown back a bit thicker, I think.

Mark Were you sick with the chemo?

Corinne Maybe a little bit while I was up there, but I was fine in between. There was no real problem. I had no setbacks or infections along the way.

Mark That's great. I've interviewed a dozen or so people and heard stories of some very hard times.

Rod We've never really had any contact with anyone, either, so we don't really know what other people go through. Probably if we'd had contact with others, especially others who have had a more dramatic time than we've had, maybe we'd have worried more. We never really knew what could happen.

Dr Marsden was being cagey. He never really told us anything. Unless you asked, then he'd tell you whatever you wanted to know. But if you didn't ask, he never told you. I suspect that was for our benefit. Too much knowledge sometimes makes you worry. We never really understood that much about Ewing's sarcoma, in particular.

Chris I think the hardest time for Corinne was actually getting back on her feet after the operations. It was hard for her to get around for quite a while. She had a lot of pain.

Mark Do you think it's changed you at all?

Corinne No, I don't think so.

Mark What do you do now?

Corinne I'm an enrolled nurse. I only finished in the middle of last year so I'm trying to get something permanent, but at the moment I'm just doing casual work.

Mark Were you always going to do that?

Corinne Not from the beginning—I wanted to be a teacher. And when I was in hospital I never wanted to be a nurse. But that changed.

Chris I think she's been changed by the experience. Having to be on the other end of the treatment and the nurses around you—both the good nurses and the bad nurses—it makes an impression.

Mark Is there anything that went on that you think could have been handled better?

Corinne No.

Rod No, it was all pretty good.

Chris One thing I noticed was that because she was

young, they were much better. Most of the time the other patients, especially when she was having the chemotherapy, were older and they weren't treated as nicely. In some cases the nurses were a bit off-hand.

Mark You were in an adult ward. At sixteen, would you have preferred to be with people your own age?

Corinne No. It never crossed my mind. It was fine at the time. While I was having the chemotherapy I liked being by myself. It was quiet and I just slept. Thinking about it now, it would have been nice to be around people my own age, but at the time it didn't worry me.

During the operations, I was in a big ward with older people, but that didn't worry me. I didn't mind.

Mark It sounds like nothing affected you. Were you told about the existence of CanTeen and groups like that?

Corinne Yes, we had a cancer support nurse came out and visited once or twice and told us about the different things we could join.

Mark Did you get involved at all.

Corinne No, I didn't. I guess I might have if it had gone on longer, but it was all over so quickly. I just went back to school and that was it.

Mark How did your friends cope?

Corinne They were a lot more worried than I was. They took it harder. They were real supportive. But they were definitely a lot more worried than I was.

Mark Did you cop anything at school, Pauline?

Pauline No. A few people used to ask how Corinne was. To be honest, I was pretty excited about it all. You know, 'my sister has cancer'. I was only fourteen, and you don't really know what's going on at that age. So I was quite excited about it. I thought it was great when she could pull her hair out. I know that sounds stupid, but that's what I thought.

Mark How did you handle it? Did you miss your Mum? Did you get jealous Corinne was getting all the attention?

Pauline I guess I got jealous. I didn't really think about it at the time, but people would come and visit and for the first ten minutes it would be 'How are you Corinne?', 'How are you Corinne?' and so on, then eventually I'd get 'Hi Pauline'. I know they didn't mean it that way, but that's how I took it at the time.

Mark But apart from that, family life just went on.

Rod Yes, everything was just so clear cut. Chemo for two days every fortnight, then the operation. Absolutely no complications.

Mark How's your leg now?

Corinne Pretty good. It gets sore now and again. I'm not sure what causes it. But overall it's pretty good.

PART 3

Body

Who, What, When and Where?

How common is it

Ewing's sarcoma is the second most common bone cancer in children, after osteosarcoma. It occurs in 2.4 out of every million children in the USA. Rates are thought to be similar among Caucasians throughout the world. It is very rare among black and Asian children.[1]

Ewing's sarcoma can strike at any age. The youngest child recorded was about four months at the time of diagnosis[2] and the oldest person was 62.[3] But it is more commonly a disease of older children; 80 per cent of cases of Ewing's sarcoma are in people under the age of twenty. The most common age for it to happen is eleven years.

It occurs equally in boys and girls up to the age of thirteen, but becomes slightly more common in boys than in girls after that age;[4] the overall ratio of males : females is 1.35 : 1. It accounts for 5–10 per cent of all bone tumours, both benign and malignant.

It occurs in only about twenty people under the age of twenty in Australia each year.[5]

It is called Ewing's sarcoma because it was first described fully by Dr James Ewing in *Proceedings of the New York Medical Society* in 1921. However the tumour had been described, without being named, in Germany as early as the 1860s.

How it behaves

A cancer is an abnormal growth of cells that is not controlled by the body's mechanisms. Usually, only just enough cells grow to replace those that are dying off, but in cancer the new cells grow faster than they are needed.

There are two main types of cancer. The most common type is carcinoma, in which the abnormal cells grow from the lining of tissues and organs. Skin cancers as well as cancers of the mouth, throat, lungs, bowel and stomach are all carcinomas.

The less common main type is the sarcoma. This is a cancer that starts off in what is called connective tissue—tissue like muscles and bones.

In Ewing's sarcoma, the cells that are growing out of control are small round cells that are not as mature as the cells normally found in bone. They seem to come from nerve tissue found in the bone. They grow rapidly and can spread into surrounding areas. Often they break away and travel through the bloodstream to lodge in different parts of the body; these are known as metastases, or secondary cancers.

Occasionally, Ewing's sarcomas grow outside the bone, in what is known as the soft tissue. This is the part of the body that is neither skin nor muscle nor bone. This type of Ewing's sarcoma is also known as an extraskeletal tumour, being outside the skeleton. This type is more common in young adults than in children.

How does it affect you?

The first thing to realise is that Ewing's sarcoma is not just a disease of the bone; it is a total body disease. While the signs of the cancer are most obvious in the one place, whether it be in the arm or leg or pelvis, there is about an 80 per cent chance that tiny deposits of the tumour have already spread throughout the body by the time the cancer appears. Because of this, treatment must involve the whole body, not just the lump.

The most common signs of a Ewing's sarcoma are pain and swelling at the site of the tumour. Of course, this doesn't help much as pain and swelling are very common in children and teenagers from all sorts of bumps and bruises, while Ewing's sarcoma is rare. Not every lump is cancer, but some are.

Just over one-quarter of people have a fever at the time of diagnosis, as well. Some people are losing weight. If the person with Ewing's is losing weight and has a fever, there is a fair chance the cancer has already spread. Ewing's sarcoma has already obviously spread by the time it is diagnosed in about 25 per cent of cases. But the fact that 80–90 per cent of people with Ewing's died before the introduction of chemotherapy, even with surgery and radiotherapy, suggests that most people have undetectable metastases at the time of diagnosis. Most commonly, it spreads to the lungs, other bones and the bone marrow. However, it can spread almost anywhere, including the spinal cord and the brain.

Ewing's sarcoma can occur in almost any bone in the body. It has been described almost everywhere, with the exception of the tiny bones in the ear.

One series of reports estimated that the most common sites for Ewing's sarcoma are:
• femur (thigh)—25%
• pelvis—14%
• tibia (shinbone)—11%

- humerus (upper arm)—10%
- fibula (small bone on outside of shin)—8%
- ribs—6%.[7]

After these come rarer sites like the bones of the hands and feet, the head and neck, and the ribs.

It can be quite difficult to find, and difficult to keep track of. For example, an eighteen-year-old man in St Louis, USA, who had Ewing's sarcoma developed a pneumothorax, a condition in which the lung pops and air escapes into the cavity around the lung. This alerted his doctors that he might have secondary cancers in his lung. They looked for them with X-rays and CAT scans which would normally find them, but nothing showed up. A month later the man had an operation to fix the pneumothorax, which kept recurring. At that time, five small nodules less than 1 cm in diameter were found.[6] Admittedly, this is a rare complication of Ewing's sarcoma, but it highlights the problems everybody faces in knowing exactly what is going on.

Long bones such as tibia, femur and humerus

If you have to have Ewing's sarcoma, it is best to have it in a long bone in a limb. And if you have to have it in a limb, it is best to have it as far away from the trunk as possible.

A tumour in a long bone is best for a number of reasons. It is usually easier to see, so it is usually found earlier. Radiotherapy is easier because it is away from vital, and easy to damage, organs. Surgery is easier because some parts of the limbs are disposable or replaceable.

This is not just commonsense. As many as 80 per cent of people with Ewing's sarcoma of the forearm or shin survive five years or more. That is a good result.

Pelvis

Tumours inside the pelvis are hard to find. They don't cause anything obvious like a lump in the arm or a swelling in the shin. They may cause a vague ache or even a severe pain, but because there is so much room in the pelvis they have usually grown quite large by the time they are diagnosed.

One study from St Bart's Hospital, and the Royal Hospital for Sick Children in London shows this clearly.[2] Thirteen out of 24 tumours of the limbs were smaller than 10 cm at the time of diagnosis, but by that stage twelve out of the sixteen Ewing's sarcomas of the pelvis had grown larger than 10 cm diameter.

They are also more likely than other tumours to have spread. In the same study, fifteen of the sixteen pelvic tumours had spread more than 2 cm into the surrounding tissue compared to twelve of the 24 limb tumours. And only two out of 24 Ewing's sarcomas of the limb had metastasised by the time of diagnosis, as had only one out of eighteen tumours on the rib. But four out of sixteen tumours in the pelvis had metastasised by the time they were diagnosed. This makes an enormous difference to their potential treatment, and to the chances of survival.

According to the US National Cancer Institute, almost half of all pelvic tumours have already metastasised by the time they are diagnosed.

A report from seven children's hospitals in Australia, USA, Italy and France shows that the average time between the onset of symptoms and diagnosis is five months.[7] The main reason for the delay is that symptoms progress slowly and are not very dramatic. They are not taken as seriously as if something had happened suddenly, or a lump had suddenly appeared. Sometimes, symptoms were ignored because there was a history of some trauma such as a fall or a knock which was thought to explain the pain.

The most common symptoms were pain, limping and a lump in the pelvis. The pain was fairly generalised in the region of the hip, groin, thigh, buttock and sometimes knee. Out of thirty patients described, only two had back pain and one had abdominal pain. But seventeen of the thirty had a lump in the abdomen which could be felt on examination.

The outlook for people with Ewing's sarcoma of the pelvis is not good. The Royal Children's Hospital in Melbourne has had only one child out of twenty survive with pelvic Ewing's[8], while other hospitals and doctors have reported that no more than 10 per cent survive.

A large group of American doctors, who have formed the Intergroup Ewing's Sarcoma Study (IESS), have been reporting their work since 1973 when chemotherapy became widely used. They compared IESS-1, which ran from 1973 to 1978, with IESS-II, which ran from 1978 to 1983.[9] They found that the survival of people with pelvic Ewing's sarcoma has improved considerably, largely due to chemotherapy, although they are still not great.

Ribs

While Ewing's sarcoma is not common in the rib, it accounted for almost 10 per cent of cases of one study looking back over forty years of the US Armed Forces.[10] Other estimates, like those above, have put it at 6 per cent of all cases of Ewing's.

Commonly people who have Ewing's sarcomas of the ribs blame some accident or injury, because that is when they are first noticed. But it is more likely that an injury causes a minute fracture in the weakened bone of the tumour, or else it causes a small bleed into the tumour which makes it suddenly swell and become noticeable.[11]

Ewing's sarcoma of the ribs tends to be picked up earlier than tumours in some other places, so the outlook tends to be better. In a small series of cases, thirteen of twenty children with Ewing's of the rib were alive at the time of reporting.

Skull

One seventeen-year-old had suffered bad headaches for two months—so bad he had been off school for the past three weeks. He had been vomiting, had hiccups and was dizzy. His balance was poor and he had to walk with his feet far apart to keep his balance. Magnetic resonance imaging (MRI, like a CAT scan) showed a large Ewing's sarcoma of his skull. A 9 cm x 7 cm section of bone was removed, then the boy had radiotherapy. Six months later, at the time the report was written, he was alive and well.[12]

But Ewing's of the skull is very rare.

Head and neck

There have been about 100 reported cases of Ewing's sarcoma of the face.[13] The average age at diagnosis is fifteen, although ages range from three to 38. Males are affected more often than females. The most common symptom is pain, which can be quite severe. Sometimes the pain is put down to dental problems, until the diagnosis becomes obvious.

It is unclear whether people with Ewing's sarcoma of the face have benefited from the improvements in treatment with the combined use of chemotherapy, radiotherapy and surgery. The last study is now 10 years old; only three out of eighteen patients had survived five years.[14] But those patients would have started treatment in 1978 at the latest, and things have changed since then.

Ewing's of the head and neck overall is not all that common. However treatment is usually effective.[15]

Skip lesion

A skip lesion is an oddity. It is a second tumour found in the same bone as the first, but the two are not connected. Between the two is normal bone and bone marrow, with no sign that the second tumour is a metastasis of the first.

Doctors are not sure how skip lesions come about. Are they just metastases? If so, why are metastases not found anywhere else in people with skip lesions? Are they a second, totally independent, tumour that just happened to start at the same time? While this explanation may seem odd, it is reasonable. Whatever induced one tumour to start up could have induced another one in the same place.

Skip lesions had been recognised for some time in osteosarcomas, but the first skip lesion in Ewing's sarcoma was not clearly described until 1989. A 22-year-old man with pain in his thigh and knee was found, on X-ray, to have an obvious tumour in his femur. There was a small oval that looked like a cyst on the X-ray just a few centimetres above the tumour, but tests seemed to rule out any chance of it being a cancer. But two months later the small cyst had grown. Further tests showed it was not a sign of spread, but definitely a skip lesion. At no time was there any sign of spread anywhere else in the body. Eventually the man had surgery to complement his chemotherapy. Three years later he appeared to be free of disease.[16]

It is possible that skip lesions are quite common, occurring in 20 per cent or more of bones with Ewing's sarcomas.[17]

Extraskeletal tumour

Extraskeletal tumours are rare. Even though they are found in the soft tissues, the cells that have turned malignant are the same as those that form the cancer in the more common bony Ewing's sarcoma. The main difference is that extraskeletal Ewing's sarcomas occur more often in young adults than in children; the average age in one series was 22.[18] However, there has been an extraskeletal Ewing's sarcoma in a girl as young as four.[19]

Extraskeletal Ewing's sarcomas are found in different sites. They are more likely to be in the chest, abdomen or pelvis, although the limbs are still common sites. There appears to be no gender predilection.[19]

About three-quarters of people with an extraskeletal Ewing's sarcoma have a lump, while about two-thirds have a pain as well. Those arising in the trunk are likely to be painful, while those in the limbs are more likely to be noticed as a painless lump.

Symptoms are not always straightforward though. Extraskeletal Ewing's sarcomas can show up in odd ways. One young girl had a blocked nose that just gradually got worse. Another girl with a tumour between her vagina and rectum had diarrhoea and a constant urge to pass urine.

Pregnancy

Ewing's sarcoma has been reported to occur in pregnant women. The babies were delivered healthy, and the women started chemotherapy soon after birth. Pregnancy did not seem to influence the women's chances of survival.[20]

What Causes
Ewing's Sarcoma?

Nobody knows what causes Ewing's sarcoma. There are many questions and many theories. Some of those described below may turn out to be accurate, some may not. At the moment it is impossible to say which is which.

But it is important to understand that with most cancers, little is known about the cause. We know smoking causes lung cancer, and sun exposure causes skin cancer. For many of the others, we know things that might increase your chances of getting cancer (like a high fat diet increases your chances of bowel cancer) but we cannot say there is a direct cause-and-effect relationship.

So Ewing's is not particularly unusual. Because it is relatively rare, not a lot of research has been done. But it is fair to say that as much is known about the causes of Ewing's as about many of the other less common cancers.

Is it height? Or growth?

There was a theory that children who grew quickly were vulnerable to Ewing's sarcoma. The theory makes sense—after all, Ewing's often occurs in teenagers who are growing rapidly, and it occurs most often in the fast-growing bones of the limbs. Some parents will tell you that the cancer appeared soon after their child's growth spurt.

The theory was kicked off in 1966 when it was reported in the American *Journal of the National Cancer Institute* that larger breeds of dogs were much more prone to getting bone sarcomas than smaller breeds.[1]

That sparked the interest of Dr Joseph Fraumeni of the US National Cancer Institute, who found that tall children were more likely to get osteosarcoma, another form of bone cancer, than small children. Ewing's sarcoma also affected more tall children, although not to the same extent.[2]

It makes sense in other ways, too. Adults who have various conditions where bone is growing faster than it normally should are prone to developing bone cancers. These conditions include infections such as osteomyelitis and hormonal conditions such as hyperparathyroidism and Paget's disease.

A research report from the US National Cancer Institute says that osteosarcoma, the other type of bone cancer in young people, definitely is related to a growth spurt.[3] But osteosarcoma is not the same as Ewing's sarcoma.

And a study of 236 children with leukaemia showed that they were, on average, much taller than other children their own age.[4] The authors suggested that a growth hormone known as somatomedin may be important in the development of the leukaemia. Even if this is true, it is unclear whether it has any relevance to Ewing's sarcoma.

Recent research has not supported the idea. One study in 1984, which checked the height of 291 children and teenagers with Ewing's sarcoma, found that boys who developed the cancer were the same size as their peers, or maybe slightly heavier, while girls who developed it were smaller than normal.[5] A study in 1987 found that children who developed any type of cancer were no taller than children who did not.[6]

If the tumour was related in some cases to puberty, then you would expect the average age of girls with Ewing's sarcoma to be lower than the average age of boys with Ewing's, as girls go through puberty a year or two earlier than boys. But this doesn't happen—girls and boys are affected by Ewing's at the same age.

In 1987 doctors from St Jude Children's Research Hospital in Memphis, Tennessee, published a review of all 3657 children admitted to the hospital between 1962 and 1985. They found no difference in height between children with and children without cancer.[6]

So with some evidence either way, but the more recent evidence going against it, doctors tend to think that the growth spurt is not related to the formation of Ewing's sarcoma. But the decision is not yet final.

Is it radiation?

The role of irradiation is hard to work out. If radiation was a cause of Ewing's sarcoma, you would expect there to have been a rise in the incidence of the cancer after the atomic bombing of Hiroshima and Nagasaki. But that did not happen (or, if it did, it was not noticed).

However children who have radiation for Ewing's sarcoma do have a slightly increased risk of developing a second Ewing's at some later stage. See a later chapter for more details on this.

Is it genetic?

Is Ewing's sarcoma passed on through some families? Are some people more prone to developing the cancer because of their family background? This question has bothered a few researchers.

Doctors have described three cases of sisters with Ewing's, and one of brothers with Ewing's. There has also been a father and daughter in Australia who both developed, and survived, Ewing's sarcoma.[7] For such a rare tumour, this seems to be more than a coincidence.

In one case, a nine-year-old girl and her nineteen-year-old sister both developed Ewing's sarcomas in their right thigh. Doctors from the Massachusetts General Hospital in Boston, USA, who treated both girls, were surprised and tried to find out whether this could be due to anything except plain bad luck.

They investigated the family; no cancers among mother, father, elder brothers, grandparents, aunts, uncles and cousins. No other serious illness in the family. No exposure of anyone in the family to radiation or known cancer-causing agents. Chromosomal studies of the girls were normal. In fact, nothing showed up. The doctors clearly didn't think it was just chance. But they could find no other explanation. Bad luck it was.[8]

British doctors have shown that mothers of children who develop osteosarcoma and chondrosarcoma, another type of sarcoma, seem to be three times as likely as the average woman to develop breast cancer.[9,10]

They then asked whether the same risk of cancer in the family existed for Ewing's sarcoma. If so, it would increase the likelihood of Ewing's having a genetic basis. They followed up 61 children with Ewing's, but found that their mothers were no more likely than the average woman to have breast cancer, or indeed any cancer. However the study was fairly small and it is possible that it was not large enough to show a true link.

Children who survive retinoblastoma, a cancer of the eye with a strong genetic link, are more likely than the average child to develop osteosarcoma and Ewing's sarcoma.

At a more scientific level, specific chromosomal abnormalities have been found. In every cell of our bodies, we have 23 pairs of chromosomes. The pairs are long strands of DNA, joined in the middle. They look something like a four-legged spider would look.

Each chromosome contains thousands and thousands of genes. This genetic material is responsible for us having brown hair, or big eyes, or buck teeth, or natural sporting ability, or natural intelligence. But many people think genes stop working once you are born. This is wrong; in fact, genes work throughout our lives influencing everything that goes on inside our bodies.

Researchers have found that something is wrong in the chromosomes of many people who develop Ewing's sarcoma. The long arms of chromosome 11 and chromosome 22 have crossed over and swapped their genetic material around. This is called a translocation (swapped location), and it happens at a particular point. Scientifically, it is described as a translocation at t(11; 22)(q24;q12). These translocations are only found in the cells of a Ewing's sarcoma. They are not found in other cells even in people with Ewing's.[11]

Exactly what this means is unclear. You *can* get Ewing's sarcoma and not have a translocation. And you can have a translocation and not get Ewing's. And that t(11; 22)(q24;q12) translocation is found in two related cancers: Askin's tumour and peripheral neuroectodermal tumour (PNT, also known as neuroepithelioma) and esthesioneuroblastoma, which is a very rare malignant tumor arising from nerves in the nasal passages.[12]

The cells of these tumours look similar to those of Ewing's sarcoma under the microscope, being small round cells, and they react similarly to many of the tests done in pathology labs. It seems likely that they come from the same original cells, and they might arise and multiply for the same reason, but nobody knows what that reason is.

To highlight the links between the two, American doctors recently described chromosomal damage in children with Ewing's sarcoma and PNT. These children had the usual t(11;22)(q24;q12) translocation, but they also had a translocation between chromosomes 1 and 16—written as der(16)t(1;16)(q21;q13). This suggests a close link between PNT and Ewing's sarcoma.

Just to confuse things further, British doctors have described the case of an eight-year-old girl with Ewing's sarcoma of the pelvis. She was found to have an abnormal chromosome number 22. But the abnormality was not the usual t(11;22)(q24;q12); it was elsewhere on chromosome 22. Chromosome 11 was not affected. The doctors suggest this may mean that chromosome 22 is more important in Ewing's than chromosome 11.[13] Backing this theory is evidence that damage to chromosome 22 has been shown to be associated with Burkitt's lymphoma and chronic myeloid leukaemia— both cancers of the immune system.

Interestingly, both Ewing's sarcoma and PNT are rare in black and Asian children. Does this mean genes are somehow important?

Was it a knock?

People who develop cancer or who have a relative with cancer will often say that it started after a broken ankle, or a heavy tackle at football, or a bump on the breast. It is difficult to say whether this is true or not. Doctors think that the most likely explanation is that bump or bruise drew attention to a sore part of the body, or that it made an underlying lump appear more obvious.

Is it something in the environment?

Californian researchers decided to try to work this one out, and interviewed the families of 43 children who had been treated for Ewing's sarcoma between 1978 and 1986.[14] Interviews covered the children's parents' occupation and exposure to chemicals at work; height and weight; use of cigarettes, alcohol and other drugs; details of the mothers' pregnancy, including exposure to drugs and X-rays; family income; family history of birth defects and cancer; and where the family lived (city or country). They carried out similar interviews with families of children of similar ages who had not developed Ewing's.

They found that seven of the 43 children who developed Ewing's sarcoma had fathers who worked in agriculture. In comparison, only five of the 193 control fathers worked in agriculture. Of the Ewing's group, two fathers were gardeners, one was a ranch foreman, two were dairy farmers and two were vegetable growers. All these fathers were working in agriculture before and at the time of conception. All reported that they were frequently exposed to herbicides, pesticides and fertilisers. In other studies, herbicides and pesticides have been associated with soft tissue sarcomas.[3]

There was also a slight association between the child's mother having taken two types of drugs during pregnancy—thyroid hormone and antibiotics.

Ewing's sarcoma was also more common in people who had taken an overdose previously—the drugs taken varied enormously and ranged from aspirin and cough syrup to Valium and vitamins to paints and rat poisons. But it is hard to see how an overdose would lead directly to the formation of a tumour.

They also found a case of two brothers with Ewing's sarcoma whose father had always worked in agriculture. The brothers, aged eight and fifteen, were diagnosed within months of each other.

How could a father's exposure to herbicides or pesticides increase the chances of his child developing Ewing's sarcoma? The Californian researchers suggested a few different mechanisms. Perhaps the father was bringing home chemicals or viruses. Perhaps agricultural chemicals affected the genetic material in the father's sperm before conception. Perhaps during pregnancy the mother was exposed to viruses or chemicals brought home from the farm. These are just educated guesses— nobody yet knows.

Is it a virus?

Viruses are associated with some cancers. For example, the human papilloma virus, or wart virus, is associated with cervical cancer in women. And the Epstein-Barr virus is associated with a type of lymphoma (a cancer of the immune system). Also, viruses have been linked with Paget's disease, which causes painful swelling of bones. Paget's disease can go on to become osteosarcoma in some people. Because of links like these, researchers have investigated whether sarcomas could be caused by a virus.

This research was spurred by findings that some viruses have caused sarcomas in experimental animals like rats and mice. As well, about twenty years ago particles that look like viruses were seen in osteosarcomas.

Two British scientists decided to test whether bone sarcomas could be caused by a virus, by seeing whether there had been an 'outbreak'. Viral infections tend to occur in a lot of people in one area at the same time, so if viruses caused Ewing's, then you would expect to find a lot of people developing Ewing's in the one area at the same time.

These scientists examined every bone sarcoma in people aged under 25 over a fifteen-year period in England. They found no evidence of outbreaks during that time; there was no congregation of cases of sarcoma in a local geographical area, nor was there any outbreak of them in any particular year.[15] A similar study in the USA in 1970 found a similar result.[16] While these studies are not definitive evidence that a virus could not be causing sarcomas, they suggest it is unlikely.

Some confusing evidence came from Western Australia in 1983.[17] Six cases of Ewing's were discovered in a two-year period, far more than normal. All were in males aged twelve to 34. All lived on or near farms most of their lives. Two men knew each other well. Doctors investigating the cluster say it is possible, though by no means likely, that these cases of Ewing's were induced by a virus or some other sort of infection.

Is it something else?

There seems to be no association with congenital diseases like rubella or Down syndrome. Some researchers have suggested that children who develop Ewing's sarcoma are more likely to have minor congenital abnormalities of the urinary system, but others have found such abnormalities to be less common in people with Ewing's.

So what is it?

We'll go back to where we started—nobody knows. Genes probably play a part. The environment probably plays a part. Exposure to radiation may play a part. Who knows what else it could be?

What Are
Our Chances?

It is the obvious question. My child has cancer—will he live? Will she die? What are our chances?

Before chemotherapy, the outlook for somebody with Ewing's sarcoma was fairly grim. Although the tumour could often be removed by either surgery or radiotherapy, it usually came back. Probably, it had already spread at the time of diagnosis, even if that spread was not obvious. Probably small numbers of cells had moved through the bloodstream but not yet grown large enough to be seen. Either that, or the radiotherapy reduced the size of the tumour but did not kill every cell. For these reasons, three decades ago only 5–10 per cent of people with Ewing's sarcoma survived more than a few years.[1]

But chemotherapy, which was introduced in the 1960s and early 1970s and has been gradually improved, has made an enormous difference. Chemotherapy is the use of strong drugs to kill cancer cells. At first, only one drug at a time was used. But now doctors are finding that combinations of two, three or even four drugs are much more effective. They allow lower doses of the drugs to be given and make resistance to the drugs, when the drugs become virtually ineffective, less likely.

Cure is now possible. Of course with cancer, doctors tend not to talk of 'cure' because of the disease's unpredictability. They talk of five-year survival—that is, being alive five years after treatment starts. While nobody can be certain that this is a cure, as occasionally Ewing's can come back even after that time, it is as close as doctors get to talk of 'cure'.

Success rates vary. It is difficult to say 'your chances of success are this or that'. To highlight the variations and results, we will go through the results from a number of different hospitals and clinics. These are world leaders in treating Ewing's sarcoma.

Two points must be made about these reports. They are based on old treatments. For example, a study published in 1990 will usually include people who were treated in 1970. The results of people being treated in 1990 will probably not be published until the year 2000. That is because it is no use saying 'the operation was a success' until you are five years or more down the track, and you are confident the cancer is unlikely to come back.

Also, they are based on aggregates of cases. So if one study says that, on average, the five-year survival of people with Ewing's sarcoma is 50 per cent, that does *not* mean your child's chances of survival are 50 per cent. It is more of an indication for other doctors so they can compare treatments and results. Every person with Ewing's is an individual whose chances of survival must be assessed individually. We are presenting them so you can see the patterns—that it is better to have no signs of spread than obvious spread, that it is better to have the cancer in your foot than your pelvis, and so on.

With those reservations in mind, here they are.

Istituto Ortopedico Rizzoli, Bologna, Italy

Doctors at the Bone Tumour Centre of the Istituto Ortopedico Rizzoli, in Bologna, Italy, reported on 144 cases of Ewing's sarcoma treated between 1972, when chemotherapy was first used, and 1982.[2] All had localised disease only—none had known metastases at the time of diagnosis. That is, there was no sign the cancer had spread.

To treat the primary tumour, ten had an amputation, 48 had lesser surgery followed by radiotherapy and 86 had radiotherapy alone. To prevent any secondary spread, all had chemotherapy. The drugs used were vincristine, doxorubicin and cyclophosphamide, while some also had dactinomycin. The chemotherapy was given intermittently over a period of two years.

Every patient responded well to the initial treatment. They felt better and the tumour got smaller. Within one to two months, the X-rays started looking better.

Fifty-nine patients (41 per cent) were completely free of disease at the time of reporting, which was between five and sixteen years after their cancer appeared. Nearly all of these could be considered cured.

Eighty-one patients (56 per cent) had a relapse—seven with a recurrence of the primary tumour, 46 with metastases and 28 with both.

Four patients (2.7 per cent) developed a second tumour—two of those are alive and well ten years after treatment.

To highlight the fact that recurrences do not always occur in the first couple of years, as with many tumours, seven people developed their recurrence or their second tumour more than five years after the primary tumour.

About 60 per cent of those who were treated by radiotherapy as well as surgery to control the primary tumour appeared to be cured, compared to only 28 per cent of those who had radiotherapy alone.

Chances of cure were improved by using four drugs in chemotherapy, rather than three drugs.

The chances of the tumour coming back in the same place varied according to the site of the primary tumour—47 per cent of pelvic tumours recurred, compared to 17 per cent in other bones of the trunk and 18 per cent in tumours of the arms and legs.

Of the 74 who developed metastases, only three were alive and well at the time of reporting (no more than four years after their metastases appeared). The rest died, an average of thirty months after the metastases appeared.

CESS-81 and CESS-86 (German Society of Paediatric Oncology)

The German Society of Paediatric Oncology asked doctors in fifty hospitals throughout Europe to study Ewing's sarcoma. The first study, CESS-81, used a combination of chemotherapy, radiotherapy and surgery. They claim 50 per cent of their patients are alive five years after diagnosis.[3]

A couple of interesting points arose from that study. One was that they re-examined the treatment of people who had suffered recurrences of the tumour after radiotherapy. They found that the radiotherapy had been incorrectly given in almost every case, so they made efforts to ensure radiotherapy was given properly through a quality assurance programme. Since that programme started, the quality of radiotherapy has improved and nobody has had a recurrence of the primary tumour after radiotherapy.

As well, as described elsewhere, the size of the tumour is important in determining the chances of survival. People with smaller tumours are more likely to survive.[1]

With CESS-86, a few changes were made. Children with large tumours were given high doses of the drug ifosfamide instead of cyclophosphamide. As well, they had surgery or radiotherapy after nine weeks of chemotherapy, rather than eighteen weeks as in CESS-81. The results were impressive, with survival rates almost doubling from 31 per cent to 61 per cent.[4]

IESS-I and IESS-II (Inter-group Ewing's sarcoma study)

In 1972 doctors throughout the United States joined together to form the Inter-group Ewing's sarcoma study, or IESS. Their work was supported, in part, by grants from the US National Cancer Institute. They have set up two studies—IESS-I from 1973–78, and IESS-II from 1978–82. They compared different forms of treatment to see what worked best. It is important to note that everybody included in the study was free of metastases at the time of diagnosis. So the survival figures don't speak for everybody with Ewing's; they speak only for those whose cancer appeared to be isolated to one place at the time they were diagnosed.

The group recently published a review of the results of IESS-I.[5] By the time of publication, all patients who survived had been alive at least six years after diagnosis, so that was a long enough period to get a fair idea of what would happen.

Patients were more likely to survive the cancer if they were younger and if their tumour was anywhere except the pelvis. Only 34 per cent of those with pelvic sarcomas survived five years, compared to 57 per cent with sarcomas elsewhere. They noted that those with pelvic tumours were more likely than those with the cancer elsewhere to die after five years, as well. Living five years is not quite long enough to call it a 'cure', especially with pelvic disease.

Almost half these patients developed metastases— commonly in either the bones or the lungs. Some of these patients had received radiotherapy to the lungs in an effort to prevent metastases happening; clearly this did not work.

Age at diagnosis proved to be important. Those aged under ten had a 71 per cent five-year survival, compared to only 46 per cent of those over fifteen at the time of diagnosis.

At the same time, they reviewed the results of IESS-II, which again was used to compare treatments for people with Ewing's sarcoma which had not metastasised at the time of diagnosis.[6,7]

They found that intermittent high dose chemotherapy was more effective than continuous moderate dose chemotherapy. The patients expressed no real preference for either.

They learnt from IESS-I that ordinary methods of treatment were not good enough for people with Ewing's in the pelvis. So they changed their approach. In IESS-II, people with pelvic Ewing's received six weeks of chemotherapy, then either surgery or radiotherapy or both, then almost eighteen months of chemotherapy. The results showed a great improvement—after five years more than half the patients appeared totally free of cancer.[7]

They feel that part of the improvement came from the advent of CAT scanning, which enables doctors to work out exactly where the tumour is and whether it has spread. They also think intermittent chemotherapy, rather than continuous chemotherapy, is more effective. In fact, the US doctors feel their results of treating people with pelvic Ewing's can be almost as good as those from treating people with Ewing's elsewhere, as long as the cancer has not spread when it is picked up. Unfortunately, this is not all that common.

National Cancer Institute

The US National Cancer Institute started using chemotherapy in 1968. Recently it reported on the results of all 107 cases of Ewing's sarcoma treated there between that date and 1980.[8]

They found that 29 per cent of people treated were free of disease after five years, and a further 10 per cent were alive but had signs of that the tumour had come back. There were a few cases of people relapsing after five years.

Note that these results are based on treatment given between 1968, when chemotherapy was first introduced, and 1980. More drugs have been added to the regimen since then, and doctors are using them more effectively. Presumably, survival rates will be higher in people treated now for Ewing's sarcoma.

Hopeful signs

- no signs of spread at diagnosis
- small tumour (less than 8 cm diameter)
- tumour in long bones of arm or leg
- tumour of hand, foot or head and neck
- no spread outside bone
- weight stable
- short duration of symptoms (less than six months)
- good response to chemotherapy

Chances of survival

Every person with Ewing's sarcoma is an individual who must be treated according to his or her specific situation. There are no blanket rules for Ewing's sarcoma, just as there are no rules for any cancer.

Having said that, there are certain things that give doctors a clue as to your child's chances of survival. Listed below are a series of factors which will make it more likely, or less likely, that your child will respond to treatment.

Metastases

Metastases are secondary cancers that have spread from the primary one.

Between 20 per cent and 30 per cent of people with Ewing's sarcoma already have detectable metastases at the time of diagnosis. Treatment for these people is much harder than treatment for people without metastases. It appears that while treatment can definitely prolong life and ease symptoms, cure is difficult. But between 10 per cent and 30 per cent with metastases at the time of diagnosis may be cured.[9]

If metastases develop during or after chemotherapy, effective treatment is harder still. The chances of cure for these people has probably dropped to less than 10 per cent.[10]

Size of tumour

The size of the tumour seems to be quite important in Ewing's sarcoma. This seems to be fairly self-evident, but it is not the case in every cancer to the same degree.

The size that most doctors estimate to make the difference is 8 cm. For example, in one study of people with Ewing's sarcoma receiving radiotherapy to the primary tumour, only two out of sixteen who had a tumour less than 8 cm diameter had a recurrence at the primary site. In contrast, nine out of sixteen with tumours larger than 8 cm had a recurrence at the primary site.[9]

In another study, 90 per cent of tumours less than 8 cm diameter went away with irradiation compared to only 52 per cent of those larger than 8 cm.[11] In another, the 3-year disease-free survival rate was 78 per cent for tumours with a volume less than 100 ml compared to 17 per cent for tumors greater than 100 ml volume.[12]

However, the size of the tumour may only be important in determining whether the primary tumour is brought under control or not. It may not be that important in working out the chances of survival. It may well be that getting the primary tumour under control is important for preventing local recurrences, which can be painful and difficult to treat, but the most important way to increase survival may be by stopping metastases through chemotherapy.

Position of tumour

It is clear that the more obvious the tumour, the better the chances of detecting it early and starting treatment early. Tumours in the limbs are likely to be much easier to see and feel than those hidden away inside the trunk. For that reason, people with tumours in the arms and legs have a better chance of survival than those with tumours of the chest or pelvis.

In one study from the US National Cancer Institute, 93 per cent of primary tumours below the knee or elbow were destroyed by radiotherapy. This proportion dropped to 67 per cent for tumours arising in the pelvis, vertebrae, ribs or breastbone. This is mainly because there is a limit to how much radiotherapy can be given to tumours in the chest or abdomen, because of the risk of damage to vital organs.

The cure rate for tumours arising either below the knee or below the elbow is probably about 60–70 per cent.[13]

Weight loss

Once somebody who has a cancer has started to lose weight, it is usually a sign the cancer has spread beyond the original tumour, or metastasised. This is probably due to proteins released by the body in response to the cancer.[14] Usually, that reduces the person's chances of survival.

Duration of symptoms

It is better to pick up the cancer early. That reduces the chances of it having spread. But it is possible to treat it as soon as a lump appears and still have metastases. Also, it is possible to ignore a lump for six months and find the cancer has not spread. It is common for the cancer to be diagnosed after symptoms of pain or a lump have been present for quite a while.

Relapse

A relapse is a recurrence of the cancer—that is, it has come back after apparently being gone. Relapses can occur after long periods of good health. They have been recorded as late as ten years after apparently successful treatment.

A relapse at the site of the original tumour is not a good sign. Survival is possible, but most people who have relapses at the site of the original tumour die within six to nine months.[3]

However there is always hope. Swedish doctors report

one patient of theirs who had surgery for a recurrence in the rib and was still well five years later, while another had radiotherapy for a secondary tumour in the brain and was alive and well eight years later.[15]

Overall

Overall, it may be wise to consider things this way. The chances of survival for the average person with Ewing's sarcoma are about 50 per cent. But no person is average, nor does anybody have the 'average' cancer. Chances will go up slightly or down slightly depending on a range of other factors. But there are no certain deaths and no certain cures. Luck plays a big part in the treatment of any cancer. All that can be done is to try your best and and hope for the best.

What Tests Will My Child Have?

Anybody who seems to have cancer will go through a number of tests to confirm the diagnosis and to see whether, or where, it has spread. These tests can be done in any order, and over any period of time, depending on the circumstances.

Full blood count (FBC)

This is a test you will get to know well. It is a simple blood test which can be done quite quickly in any pathology lab. It shows how many red cells, white cells and platelets are in your blood. Red cells are responsible for carrying oxygen, white cells for fighting infection and platelets for helping your blood clot.

It also gives information which can help doctors decide if, for example, anaemia (low red blood cells) is due to iron depletion or vitamin B1 depletion or the chemotherapy. It can suggest whether a low white cell count is due to a viral infection or the chemotherapy.

Anybody having chemotherapy will have repeated blood counts.

ESR

The ESR is the erythrocyte (red cell) sedimentation rate. A thin tube of blood is suspended, and the lab technicians measure how far the cells settle in one hour. The measurement is given in millimetres.

Nobody really knows why, but the ESR is dramatically raised in a few conditions, one of which is cancer. The ESR is raised in about 50–60 per cent of people diagnosed with Ewing's sarcoma.[1]

Serum LDH

LDH, or lactate dehydrogenase, is an enzyme produced in the liver. It is raised in about 40 per cent of people who develop Ewing's sarcoma, and may be a sign that the cancer has spread.[1]

LDH may be able to give some clue as to your child's chances of survival. Studies have shown that people who have a high LDH level are more likely to relapse than those who don't,[2] and that normal levels mean a recurrence is unlikely.[3]

X-rays

An X-ray of the tumour usually shows a patchy moth-eaten looking bone. The tumour tends to destroy the bone it grows in. Sometimes the X-rays will show what is called an 'onion-skin' appearance. This happens when the tumour pushes on to the outer lining of the bone, forcing it out. Sometimes the X-ray will show that the tumour is growing into the surrounding soft tissues, as well.

X-rays are not perfect though. Sometimes tumours can be quite large and not show up on X-ray. And it can be very difficult to tell a cyst from a tumour. For this reason, X-rays usually do not provide enough information on their own. More tests are usually needed to find out exactly how big the cancer has grown.

Bone scan

A bone scan is a specialised X-ray involving a radioactive dye. The dye is injected into a vein, from where it travels throughout the body and accumulates in bone. It is especially attracted to bone with a very active metabolism, such as bone that contains a cancer or an infection. So the radioactive dye shows up on X-rays, and any bone cancers are highlighted.

Computer-assisted tomography (CAT) scan

(Tomography is, roughly speaking, X-rays of precise slices or sections.) A CAT scan is a series of X-rays taken from the one machine during one session of 10 to 30 minutes. It provides a three-dimensional picture of the internal organs of the body, as well as the bones. It is very good at checking the size and possible spread of tumours.

Magnetic resonance imaging (MRI)

In a way, an MRI machine is an upmarket CAT scanner. They are only available in some hospitals, but it does not use X-rays.

It is thought to be a more accurate way of assessing the state of some tumours than an examination by your doctors,[4] and it gives a slightly better picture than either CAT scan or plain X-rays in determining the extent of soft tissue involvement.[5]

It is probably the best single method of evaluating and following up a Ewing's sarcoma.[5]

Biopsy

A biopsy is a procedure in which a sample of tissue is taken from the cancer and examined under a microscope. It is impossible to diagnose Ewing's sarcoma without a biopsy. In most cases, the doctors will not know whether the lump is benign or malignant. And even if they are certain that it is malignant, they will not know what type of cancer it is until they do a biopsy. It is vitally important to know exactly what type of cancer it is, as treatment varies enormously between different types. A biopsy is indispensable.

Even so, if the doctors are suspicious that this may be a cancer, it is sometimes wise to do all the other tests first, such as X-rays, CAT scans, bone scans and so on. The reason for this is to get an idea of the size of the cancer, and whether it has spread or not. Depending on these results, the biopsy might involve taking just a small part of the tumour to see what it is, or it might involve removing the whole tumour first time.

Ideally, the biopsy should be taken from any soft tissue part of the tumour. This is better than taking it from bone, because of the risk of weakening the bone and leaving it susceptible to fracture. But if bone is all there is, then bone it is.

The biopsy site should be chosen carefully. It should not be too close to important nerves or arteries, and it should not be in a site which may be needed for a skin flap, if surgery or even amputation is eventually needed.

There are two main ways of taking a biopsy. One is to take your child to the operating theatre for a biopsy under general anaesthetic. The other way is a fine needle aspiration biopsy. This is a technique commonly used to diagnose other lumps and bumps, such as those in the thyroid. Just recently, some doctors overseas have started to use it to diagnose lumps in bone or soft tissue which they suspect could be cancer. They say it is an accurate, inexpensive and rapid test.[6]

If your child has a fine needle aspiration, it will probably be done in the doctor's surgery. Cool antiseptic will be applied to the site of your child's lump, then drapes will be put around to keep the area sterile. Your doctor will then push a very fine needle into the lump and pull out a minute piece of tissue, which will be sent to a pathologist for examination.

The whole procedure takes only a couple of minutes. It is as easy as having a blood test. The needle is so fine that no local anaesthetic is needed. It is said to be uncomfortable, but not painful.[7]

Genetic tests

In some hospitals, people with Ewing's sarcoma have blood taken for genetic examination. As explained earlier most people with Ewing's sarcoma have a specific change to their chromosomes. This change may be an important trigger of whatever process leads to the formation of cancer. If doctors can get some genetic samples from everybody with Ewing's sarcoma, their chances of learning what causes it will increase.[8]

Bone marrow aspiration

Some people with Ewing's sarcoma may have a bone marrow aspiration. This test is done to see if the cancer has spread into the bone marrow, where blood is made.

The test is not a comfortable one. It is usually done in

the ward, under local anaesthetic, although small children may have sedation or a general anaesthetic. A doctor has to put a needle through the bone in your child's hip or breastbone into the bone marrow, then pull out some of the tissue there. It does not take a long time, only ten minutes or so. But sometimes it is quite painful.

Which Treatment, and When?

What treatments are available?

There are three types of treatment available: chemotherapy, radiotherapy and surgery.

The chemotherapy, is aimed at getting rid of all the cancer cells in the body, no matter where they are.

The other two treatments, surgery and radiotherapy, are aimed at getting rid of the cancer where it was first found. This is known as the primary site. It is important to get rid of the primary cancer, because the chances of the cancer spreading increase as long as the primary cancer is still there.

It is impossible to describe exactly what form of treatment somebody with Ewing's sarcoma will be offered. Because Ewing's is relatively rare, very few doctors in the world have enough experience to be confident that what they are doing is the best treatment possible. As well, new drugs are being developed all the time that are worth trying. Obviously, the overall cure rate of 50 per cent with Ewing's sarcoma means that treatment is not perfect.

Which comes first?

When treatment involves three separate strands—chemotherapy, radiotherapy and surgery—there is an obvious question: which comes first?

Should the person with Ewing's sarcoma have surgery first, followed by radiotherapy then chemotherapy to wipe out any secondary cancers? Or should the chemotherapy come first to knock out any tiny secondary cancers before they get the chance to grow?

On the whole, most doctors believe the best chances of success come from having chemotherapy first, followed by either radiotherapy or surgery or both.[1] This is because it seems that cancer cells are scattered throughout the body at the time of diagnosis in about 80 per cent of cases.

Chemotherapy as the first line of treatment reduces the chances of the tumour metastasising. It also reduces the size of the tumour for the next form of treatment, whether it be surgery or radiotherapy. In either case, a smaller tumour is easier to treat than a larger tumour.

In Australia, the usual situation is that people with Ewing's have a course of chemotherapy for about nine weeks, then a two-week break, then a further nine weeks of chemotherapy. Then they are assessed with a full range of tests.[2] After that anything can happen.

If it seems the chemo is working well, and surgery is possible, then surgery is probably the next step. If chemo is working well but surgery is not possible, then they may have radiotherapy or may keep up the chemo. If chemo is working, but not well enough, they may have a further twenty weeks, then see if surgery is possible.

If they do have surgery, and it seems that not all the tumour was removed, then it is likely they will have radiotherapy then more chemotherapy.

That is the general idea. Usually, chemotherapy comes first, followed by whatever suits the situation best.

However a dissenting voice comes from Italian doctors who argue there is not enough evidence to think chemotherapy first up is any better than starting with surgery or radiotherapy.[3]

Why does treatment sometimes fail?

Why is it that people who have radiotherapy alone are likely to get metastases? Why does it seem important to surgically remove the primary tumour?

Doctors from the Istituto Ortopedico Rizzoli in Bologna, Italy, found that when a Ewing's sarcoma recurs, it nearly always does so right in the centre of the previous tumour. They think that this happens because some of the cells in the centre of the primary Ewing's sarcoma were nearly dead at the time of treatment. Because they get little blood supply and little oxygen, they are quite resistant to chemotherapy and radiotherapy. Ironically it is the healthier cancer cells at the outside of the tumour that are most sensitive to treatment. The near-dead ones are not affected by treatment. So some time later, when the primary tumour has shrunk away and blood is flowing back to the centre of the region, these near-dead cells revive and start growing again. The tumour comes back.

These doctors think that surgery should be used more often, even if not all the tumour can be removed. At least removing a large part of the tumour will allow radiotherapy and chemotherapy to be more effective.[4] However, other doctors disagree and think surgery should not be used too often.

What works best?

Chemotherapy is essential. Surgery or radiotherapy, or both, without chemotherapy is just not good enough.

And it seems that, in most cases, the chances of a cure are increased by the use of all three forms of treatment.

The doctors responsible for care of the person with Ewing's will formulate a plan. Make sure they discuss it with you, and explain why they want to do things in that particular order. Make sure you understand what the doctors are saying. Go back and see them again if necessary. Perhaps you could take notes or tape record your conversation, so you can listen again later. Take your partner, or a friend. Talk to your doctors, air your worries and make a joint decision.

See the following chapters for more details on chemotherapy, radiotherapy and surgery.

Who decides?

In an ideal world, you and your child would decide what to do after being given all the information you need and want. But this is not an ideal world; some doctors don't enjoy allowing their patients to have much of a say, while many people do not want to take the responsibility that goes with deciding. And sometimes there appear to be few alternatives. As well, it is hard to think clearly and make rational decisions when your child has just been diagnosed with cancer.

So usually the doctors decide, at least in the early stages. You will have to get used to seeing a lot of doctors. The primary responsibility for your child will probably fall to an oncologist, who is a specialist in cancer medicine. He or she will almost certainly work with two other specialists, a surgeon and a radiation oncologist (he or she plans and gives the radiotherapy). As well, the team that will be looking after your child will include registered nurses who specialise in children's health or cancer medicine, social workers and perhaps psychologists and child therapists. Caring for somebody with cancer, especially a child or teenager, requires a team approach. No one person has all the skills required to do it properly on their own.

What about any other medications?

If your child is taking any other pills, medicines, tablets, capsules, tonics or injections, tell your specialist about them before you start any form of treatment. Take along a list of everything your child takes, including anything just taken sometimes, like vitamins or aspirin. Ask if it is OK to keep taking them, and whether there is anything your child should not take.

While having chemotherapy, ask your specialist before you start taking any new drugs. Some chemotherapy drugs don't mix well with some other medicines.

How much will it cost?

If you don't have private health insurance, your child can be treated under Medicare. This means that you won't have to pay for any tests or treatment given at a public hospital or outpatient clinic. And you won't have to pay for your hospital bed or room.

If you want your child to be a private patient at either a public or private hospital, you will have to pay some or all of the costs. If you have private health insurance, your health fund will pay for part or most of these costs. Check with your health fund, hospital, clinic and specialists exactly how much you will have to pay yourself.

For information about health insurance or sickness benefits, or help with travel and accommodation costs, ask the hospital social worker.

What if my child refuses treatment?

Many teenagers develop a real dread of chemotherapy, and occasionally radiotherapy, because of the way it makes them feel. It is common for teenagers to develop all sorts of ruses and tricks to avoid treatment, sometimes including downright refusal to go on with it.

This raises a difficult issue. There is almost no chance of a cure without treatment. But there is no guarantee of a cure with treatment. While some people who go through chemotherapy will undoubtedly benefit, others will not. And it is not the doctor, nor the mother, nor the father, nor the brother, sister, friend nor nurse who has to put up with the side effects of chemotherapy. It is the person with the cancer, and it is well within the rights of any sane, mature person to refuse to have treatment.

The question is, at what age does a person become mature enough to decide for himself or herself? Again, there is no easy answer. Some are obviously mature enough to make important decisions at fourteen or fifteen or even younger, while others only really reach independence in their thirties. It is a question for each person, and family, to decide for themselves.

It seems fair to take this approach. Try to work out exactly what is bothering the person having, or refusing to have, the chemotherapy. Is it the nausea? Is it the loss of hair? Is it the trips to hospital? The time away from school? The fear of the unknown? The uncertainty of the situation? The fear of the drips? The tiredness? The weight loss? The hospital staff?

Listen to the concerns, and try to work out exactly what is the problem. Seen in separate parts, many of the problems of chemotherapy can be addressed, if not dealt with completely. For example, one person may fear the hair loss. While nothing can change that, using a wig or getting a range of hats or having the teenager's best friend shave his or her head in sympathy may be the trick needed to overcome that fear of being different. If it is nausea, then a change of diet or the addition of extra anti-nausea drugs may do the trick. If it is the hospital setting, then it may be possible to have treatment in a different room in the ward, or in a different part of the hospital, or given by different staff.

But in the end, if the person with the cancer decides the chances of cure are not worth all the troubles of treatment, then that is within his or her rights. Nobody should be able to force another person to go through painful treatment.

What if we want a second opinion?

It is possible that you and your child do not like one of your doctors. You might have a personality clash. Or you might not trust him or her. Or, faced with such an important event, you simply want another opinion.

It is always possible for you to seek a second opinion or even to swap doctors. The simplest way to go about it is to be honest—tell your doctor you would like a second opinion. Your doctor should be able to arrange that within the hospital, or sometimes in another hospital.

If your doctor does not agree, then you can go back to your general practitioner and ask for an urgent referral to another cancer specialist for a second opinion.

If you feel you would like to change doctors, talk to your doctor first. Explain why. Is it because you are not being told enough? Or too much? Or you don't like his or her bedside manner? Or is it something else? Sometimes talking about it will help solve the problem.

But if that does not solve the problem, then your doctor has a responsibility to refer you to another specialist as quickly as possible.

Chemotherapy

Chemotherapy is a form of treatment which uses drugs and medications to either cure or control the cancer. 'Chemo' means drugs or medicines and 'therapy' means treatment. Chemotherapy drugs are often called cytotoxic drugs—'cyto' means cells and 'toxic' means capable of killing cells.

Chemotherapy works by stopping cells from growing. Your child's body, like yours, is made up of billions of cells. Most of these cells are replaced regularly when they are worn out or old or damaged.

Some cells, like those in bones, replace themselves very slowly. Others, like those in the mouth and in hair, replace themselves very quickly. Cancer cells grow even faster than those.

The drugs work by attacking cells when they are at their most vulnerable—the stage of division and multiplication. Because fast-growing cells divide and multiply more often than slow-growing cells, fast-growing cells are more susceptible to chemotherapy than slow-growing ones. But unfortunately, chemotherapy cannot be localised to treat only the cancer cells. It attacks all cells. So every cell is affected to some degree, the faster-growing ones like cells of the hair and mouth more than the slower ones.

But because chemotherapy attacks every cell, it can kill cancer cells that cannot be seen but which could grow and become dangerous if left untreated. Chemotherapy aims to rid the whole body, not just the affected part, of cancer.

Will chemotherapy cure my child?

This is a very common question, with no easy answers. Chemotherapy can cure some types of cancer. Sometimes it can do this on its own—sometimes it does it when used together with surgery or radiotherapy.

At other times, chemotherapy is used to control cancer by stopping it growing or by making it shrink. This can give your child a longer life or can help reduce any problems the cancer is causing.

It is important, when discussing chemotherapy, to get something clear in your mind. Are you aiming for a cure? Or are you aiming to buy some time, or to control symptoms such as pain? All of the options are valid, and chemotherapy can be used successfully even when not aiming for a cure, but it is important to know what you are trying to achieve before you start.

How is chemotherapy given?

Chemotherapy can be given in one of four ways:
• By mouth—as tablets, liquids or capsules.
• By injection—into a muscle, under the skin or into a vein.
• Through an intravenous drip—a bag hung on a pole is connected to a narrow piece of tubing which carries the fluid via a needle into a vein in your child's arm.
• Via a Hickmann's catheter—this is a small catheter put into the chest under general anaesthetic, which carries drugs straight into the heart. If put in properly and looked after well, a Hickmann's catheter can last many,

many months, greatly reducing the need for drips and injections.

Most chemotherapy is given by injection or through a drip or Hickmann's catheter, although your child might be given tablets to take as well. Often these can be taken at home. Even more than most drugs, these need to be taken exactly when and how your doctor says. If you are not sure, ask your doctor to write down instructions. Or you could ring and check with the chemotherapy sister or clinic.

How long will the treatment last?

Treatment often lasts for six to eighteen months, or even longer. The average time of treatment is twelve months. It usually goes in cycles—your child gets treatment once or over a few days then has a rest before the next treatment. This gives your child a chance to recover from any side effects.

A typical approach, although by no means the only approach, is to start with either radiotherapy or chemo-therapy to the cancer. Once that is over, it is common to start chemotherapy every month or six weeks for twelve months. This chemotherapy is known as adjuvant chemotherapy.

Some doctors are trying a form of treatment known as neoadjuvant chemotherapy. With this treatment, your child would start with six weeks to two months of chemotherapy, then have a break to have radiotherapy or surgery (or both). Then the chemotherapy would resume, to make a total of sixteen months of treatment.

Which drugs will my child have?

When chemotherapy first became available in the late 1960s, doctors tried using a single drug. However they found that after a while, the drugs stopped working in some people. The cancer cells became resistant to them. Somehow the cells learnt what the drug was trying to do, and evolved a way of surviving the onslaught.

It is now clear that using more than one drug decreases the chances of resistance developing. A cell that can survive one drug may still be susceptible to another. Also, by using combinations of drugs that act in different ways, cells are more likely to be killed than by a drug acting only in one way.

The main drugs used in chemotherapy for Ewing's sarcoma are vincristine, cyclophosphamide, and dactinomycin. Others used include methotrexate, bleomycin and VP-16. More recently, another drug called doxorubicin (or Adriamycin) which can be quite effective but has serious side effects was added. It causes cardiomyopathy, a weakening of the heart, in almost 50 per cent of cases.[1] Then just in the past few years doctors have started to use new drugs called etoposide and ifosfamide. The chances are high that your doctor will use a combination of some or all of these drugs.

All of them are quite toxic. They can all cause similar side effects, then they all have their own specialised side effects peculiar to that drug. When we come to the section on side effects, we will run through the general side effects first, then list the particular ones.

Blood tests

Usually before you have each treatment a nurse or doctor takes some blood and sends it to the hospital laboratory for a blood count. This measures the levels of different types of cells in your child's blood. Blood counts are needed because chemotherapy is likely to lower the levels of these cells in your blood. For more details, see the section on tests on pages 244–5.

Does chemotherapy hurt?

Chemotherapy usually does not hurt. Tablets are just like any other tablets. Injections are just like any other injection. An intravenous drip will sting when the needle goes in, but then the pain should stop. But some of the drugs do make your child feel sick. See page 265 for possible side effects and what to do about them.

Should my child try a new drug?

Your doctor may ask you to help try a new drug. Doctors can only find new and better drugs by testing them on people. These are called clinical trials. Your child can not be in a clinical trial without your permission.

In most clinical trials some people will be getting the new drug and others will be getting older drugs that the doctors are accustomed to using. This is so they can compare the two, and see whether the new drug is any better than the old.

If your doctor asks you for permission to put your child in a clinical trial, ask him or her what the chances are of getting the new drug. Ask what the other drug is. Ask if you will know what your child is getting. Ask whether your doctor will know what your child is getting.

Find out more about the new drug. Has it been used before? What are its side effects? Why is your doctor trying it out?

Remember that your child does not have to be involved

in a clinical trial. And if you do get involved and change your mind, you are allowed to pull out of it.

What about a bone marrow transplant?

Doctors in the United States frequently use a technique known as autologous bone marrow transplantation (ABMT). It is a technique which allows higher doses of chemotherapy to be given in the hope of killing off all cancer cells in the body.

The idea is that the person with cancer undergoes a few courses of fairly mild chemotherapy, then some bone marrow is drained out of his or her hip and sternum. This is stored.

Then massive doses of chemotherapy can be given. These toxic drugs, as expected, kill off all the cells in the bone marrow. The person becomes anaemic, susceptible to infections because of a lack of white blood cells, and prone to bleed easily because of a lack of platelets.

At that stage, doctors put back the bone marrow, which has been stored and is unharmed by the chemotherapy. The cells start doing their job and recovery is fairly prompt.

While this sounds a great idea, problems exist. The higher dose chemotherapy may make little difference. Or the person might suffer serious infections before the bone marrow is transfused back.

Autologous bone marrow transplantation has been quite successful in the treatment of some forms of leukaemia, but it has not been used as often, or as successfully, in other types of cancer.

For these reasons, Australian doctors have not been as ready to undertake what they still consider an experimental procedure. They have tried bone marrow transplants, but have not been happy with the results.[2]

A study by doctors at the US National Cancer Institute

attempted to see whether there was any benefit from ABMT, high dose chemotherapy and giving a small dose of radiotherapy to the entire body.[3] The idea behind giving total body irradiation was that Ewing's sarcomas are sensitive to radiation, so giving radiation everywhere would kill any cells lurking around the body.

This combined treatment was only given to patients thought to be at high risk of dying of Ewing's—they either had metastases when they were diagnosed or their primary tumour was in a position where a cure was to be hoped for rather than expected, such as the pelvis.

As with other studies,[4,5] the results were not an overwhelming success. The cure rate for those who had metastases when they were diagnosed was low, as low as it is for other forms of treatment. And the cure rate for those without metastases was about the same as for those people who undergo less traumatic treatments than high dose chemotherapy, bone marrow transplntation and total body irradiation.

In all, neither autologous bone marrow transplantation nor total body irradiation seem to add a lot to the treatment of Ewing's sarcoma for most people. However, it is hard to generalise. There may be some circumstances where your doctors recommend the treatment.

Will my child have to stay in hospital?

Most people can have their treatment as an outpatient, living at home and only going to the hospital for each treatment.

Usually each treatment takes a few hours. First comes the blood test, then waiting for results to be sure it is OK to have the treatment. Some people stay in hospital most of the day, or overnight. Others stay in hospital for much of their treatment. If your child is having VP-16 or etoposide, he or she will have to stay in for the five-day cycle.

Some hospitals offer accommodation for families of children who live far away. Or they have arrangements with local cancer councils. Ask the doctors, nurses or social workers if you need accommodation or help with paying for it.

How will we know if the treatment is working?

It can be quite difficult to know whether or not chemotherapy is working.

The effectiveness of the treatment has nothing to do with how many side effects your child gets. Lots of side effects does not necessarily mean your child is getting any better or any worse. If your child has no side effects, it does not mean the treatment is not working, either.

Your child is likely to feel worse before feeling better. Again this does not mean that the treatment is or is not working.

Often only your doctors can say whether the chemotherapy is getting rid of the cancer or not. They do this by talking to you and your child, examining him or her and carrying out blood tests, scans and so on. Sometimes it is necessary to have lots of tests during treatment to see how the cancer is going.

While the most obvious ways to do it include simple questions like 'how are you feeling', a physical examination and some straightforward blood tests, it is clear that tumours can be tricky. Cancerous cells can be growing quite quickly, yet not be detected by the usual methods.

If your child is having chemotherapy in an attempt to cure the cancer, it is difficult to tell whether all the cancer cells have been destroyed. So you can say that if it has not come back in five or ten years, then it is not very likely to come back.

Side effects

Some people have no side effects at all. Most have one or more side effects. Occasionally, people have such severe side effects they have to stop the treatment for a while to recover. It depends on what drugs are used, what dose is used and what effect they have.

Most side effects are only temporary. They go away not too long after the treatment stops and they usually go away between treatments. But some side effects are permanent. Ask your specialist about the risk of permanent effects.

Here is a list of the more common side effects, and ways you can help your child deal with them. He or she probably won't get all of them. But tell your doctor or nurse about any side effects that do occur. They need to know how your child's body is coping with the drugs. They may be able to help control the side effects, or they may want to change the treatment to try to avoid them.

Feeling tired

Your child may feel very tired. Sometimes the tiredness lasts for a few weeks after the treatment has ended. This can be because of the treatment itself, or the cancer, or because of the travelling to the hospital and disruption to daily life.

If this happens, your child should take things easier. Do less than normal. Try doing easier, quieter things. Only do what he or she feels comfortable doing. Don't push. Rest often.

If your child isn't sleeping well, tell your doctor or

nurse. They may be able to help. But don't give any pills or medications unless they say you can.

Infections

Because chemotherapy frequently impairs the production of cells in the bone marrow, your child may end up with too few white blood cells. This will leave him or her prone to infections. The difficulty is that not only is he or she prone to infections, but he or she will find it difficult to fight them. This is likely to occur at particular times during the treatment programme.

The most common signs of an infection are these:
• high temperature (38 degrees or more Centigrade, or 100 degrees or more Fahrenheit)
• chills or constant shivering
• sweating, especially at night
• burning feeling when urinating
• severe cough or sore throat
• diarrhoea
• vomiting
• or, your child just feels very unwell.

If your child seems to have an infection, you must phone your hospital doctor or the hospital immediately. He or she needs urgent attention. Don't use aspirin or any other painkiller or medicine, unless the doctor says you can.

A new drug called Neupogen has been released on to the market. It stimulates the bone marrow to produce more white blood cells. Although it has not been around for very long, it looks as though Neupogen can reduce the severity and frequency of infections.

Anaemia

Your child is anaemic if he or she has too few red cells in the blood. This occurs for the same reasons as low white cells. Anaemia makes your child pale and tired. Severe anaemia can be dangerous, putting great strain on the heart.

It can be quite difficult to know whether your child is truly anaemic or is run down from the chemo and the cancer and everything else that is going on. The only way to really know is to do a blood test.

If your child is anaemic, several things may happen. The next cycle of chemotherapy may be delayed until the blood count comes back to normal. He or she may be put on iron tablets to build up the blood. Or a blood transfusion may be suggested.

Easy bruising and bleeding

Rarely, chemotherapy can interfere with the production of the cells which allow blood to clot, the platelets. Problems with low platelets can show up as large bruises from small knocks, or multiple tiny bruises which look like a rash, or bleeding noses for no reason, or blood in the urine or bowel. If any of these happen, you should contact your doctor.

Similar options apply as for anaemia—the next treatment cycle may be delayed until the platelet count comes back to normal, or a transfusion of platelets may be suggested.

Feeling sick or vomiting

Nausea and vomiting are common problems for people having chemotherapy. See pages 312–13 for details on what to do.

Not wanting to eat

Some people have no problems with their appetite during treatment. Others find they don't feel like eating.

Or they find their sense of taste changes. This can be because of the treatment, their cancer or just because of the whole experience of having cancer and being treated for it.

It is best for your child to try to eat as well as possible during treatment to maintain strength. If your child doesn't feel like eating, try different foods until you find foods he or she wants to eat. Give smaller amounts more often. Or try drinking special liquid foods which you can get from your pharmacist.

Most cancer councils have booklets and information you might find helpful. Or the hospital may have its own diet information for cancer patients. You can also talk to the hospital dietitian for advice.

Losing hair or going bald

Because of the drugs used, everybody being treated for Ewing's sarcoma in Australia will lose their hair. Hair might fall out soon after the first treatment or it may not fall out for quite a while. But when it does fall out, it is likely to fall out quite quickly. Your child's scalp may feel hot or itchy just before it starts to fall out.

If your child does lose hair, it will usually grow back again when treatment stops. It takes between four and twelve months to grow back a full head of hair. It may not be as thick as it was before. It can be a slightly different colour. Or it may be finer or curlier than it was before. It can be quite itchy while it is growing back. Frequent shampooing can help the itching. Occasionally after chemotherapy, the hair doesn't grow back properly. Instead it grows back patchily.

Many people find losing their head hair very upsetting. Others don't. Try to remember that it will almost certainly grow back again.

Until it does grow back, your child has a few options. He or she can wear a wig to cover up baldness or patchiness. If this suits, it is a good idea to get a wig fitted before your child starts losing hair, so it is ready when it does fall out. Also, this makes it easier to match the colour.

Many hospitals have a wig bank or library. You may be able to borrow a free wig from them. Or if you are on a low income you may be able to get a free wig under special government schemes. Some support groups have wig banks or libraries too. If you want to buy one, expect to pay between $100 and $600 for a synthetic one, and around $1000 for one made out of real hair. And note that wigs made of real hair can take more time and money to look after than synthetic ones. If you are in a private health fund, you may be able to get some of this cost back (but check with the fund before you buy). Ask your doctor, nurse or the hospital social worker for more information about how to go about getting free wigs or where to buy them.

Some people don't bother with a wig—they stay bald, or cover up with a scarf or hat. A bald head can be a fashion statement, especially for a child or teenager who would like to look a bit different. It's up to your child. There is no medical reason why a wig is necessary, and it is far better to be happy and bald than self-conscious about a wig.

The only thing about going bald is that your child's scalp will be more sensitive to the sun than usual. He or she should wear a hat or a high protection suncream (SPF 15+) when in the sun.

Sore or dry mouth or throat

Chemotherapy can cause a sore mouth or mouth ulcers because it damages cells that replace themselves quickly, as these ones do.

It is wise to keep teeth, gums and mouth very clean during treatment to help stop infections. The nurses can show you how to do this. Your child should use a very soft toothbrush or a cotton bud for teeth and gums, or brush his or her teeth with fingers, rather than a toothbrush.

Your specialists may supply a special liquid mouthwash to use for a red or sore mouth. You can make one yourself by mixing 1 teaspoon of salt, 1 teaspoon of baking soda (sodium bicarbonate) in 1200 ml of warm water. Use it three times a day after meals. Don't use a commercial mouthwash.

Your child should eat soft foods and drink plenty of fluids, but not anything with a high acid level such as grapefruit, tomato or orange. Spicy foods and any particular food or drink that stings should be avoided. If it does, don't eat it. A lip salve or ointment on the lips can help stop them drying out.

If your child is having trouble swallowing because of a sore and dry mouth or throat, try some of these ideas:
• suck on ice blocks
• drink lots of liquids
• moisten foods with butter
• dunk biscuits in tea
• blend foods
• eat soups and ice creams
• ask your dentist, doctor or nurse about artificial saliva
• avoid cigarette smoke.

Itchy skin and other skin problems

Your child's skin may go red; it may peel or it may become dry and itchy. Acne may develop or worsen.

Always tell your doctor about any skin problems. Try dusting cornflour over the itchy parts. Use a lotion or cream to stop the dryness. Ask your doctor for something to help if these suggestions don't work.

It is a good idea for your child to cover up and use a high protection suncream (SPF 15+) when having chemotherapy. Or just keep it out of the sun. Many of the drugs can make skin much more sensitive to the sun than it was before.

Bowel or urine problems

Sometimes people get diarrhoea from chemotherapy. If this happens, here are a few suggestions for your child:
• eat warm or cold rather than hot foods
• add low fibre foods such as bananas or macaroni to your diet
• don't eat high fibre foods like raw fruits, vegetables and bread
• drink lots of liquid to replace the fluid you are losing
• eat smaller amounts of food more often
• don't eat foods like cabbage, fizzy drinks, highly spiced food or beans that can cause cramp
• don't eat dairy foods like milk or cheese.
If it lasts longer than 24 hours, tell your doctor.

Sometimes people become constipated from chemotherapy (and/or painkillers). Here are a few suggestions:

• drink lots of fluid
• eat high fibre foods such as nuts, raw fruits and vegetables, whole grain breads and cereals. For example, add bran to breakfast cereal.
If this doesn't work, ask your doctor for something to help. Do not leave it go too long before you try to do something about it.

The drugs may make your child's urine go a different colour or smell odd. If this happens, tell your doctor or nurse.

Stunted growth?

Children who have chemotherapy often do not grow very much during their treatment. But it seems that they catch up reasonably well and finish close to, although possibly a couple of centimetres less than, the height they would have been without treatment.[6]

Swelling or puffiness

Your child may get swollen or puffy feet, hands, stomach or face. Ask your doctor what to do about this. It is possible fluid is being retained. Your child may need to change his or her diet. Or your doctor may give something to help. Or he or she may change the treatment altogether.

Feeling depressed, down or nervous

Some people find the treatment difficult to deal with. It can seem to go on forever. It can be difficult to know whether your child is getting better or worse. If this is what is worrying you, ask your specialist how things are going.

Going to the hospital for the treatment may make your child, or anyone else in your family, depressed or nervous. For example, it is common for people to feel hopeful when their treatment begins, down in the first few weeks, up half way through, down again a little later on and depressed when their treatment ends. Your child may follow this pattern or may not. There is no right or wrong way to feel. But it is always best to try to be as hopeful and positive as possible. Remember that many people are alive and well years after finishing their chemotherapy treatment.

It is a good idea to talk to your child about his or her feelings whenever possible. Many children feel their parents are not honest with them, and are scared that something else is going on that they do not know about. Remember that you do not have cancer—your child does.

You should also talk about your own feelings to your child, your partner, family or friends. Talking often helps. If you don't feel like talking with people who are close to you, you can talk to the hospital social worker or nurse. Or you may want to talk to people who have been through the same sort of experience as you. Ask your nurse or hospital social worker about how to get in touch with someone who has been through the same sort of experience.

Other side effects

The truth is that chemotherapy can cause almost any side effect. People who are having chemotherapy are more likely than the average person to develop tuberculosis, herpes, kidney disease, viral infections of the brain, pneumonia and a multitude of other problems.

All of these are extremely rare, but they can happen. The commonsense approach is to not worry about rarities in advance, but to make sure your child is checked out by a doctor every time he or she is unwell.

Side effects from specific drugs

The main drugs used are cyclophosphamide, vincristine, and dactinomycin. Others used include methotrexate and bleomycin. More recently, another drug called doxorubicin which can be quite effective but has serious side effects was added. It causes cardiomyopathy in almost 50 per cent of cases.[1] Just in the past few years doctors have started to use new drugs called etoposide and ifosfamide.

Dactinomycin

Also known as actinomycin-D. If given after irradiation, it can cause a skin reaction that outlines where the radiation was given for months or even years. This is called the 'recall phenomenon'.

As well, it can affect the heart. An 8-year-old boy was admitted to hospital in Pavia, Italy, with a Ewing's tumour the size of an orange in his groin. He was cured by radiotherapy, chemotherapy and surgery.

But 25 months after treatment started, he developed severe heart disease. This was thought to be due to doxorubicin, one of the chemotherapy drugs he had been given. His condition deteriorated and four months later, at the age of ten years and four months, he had a heart transplant. Twelve months later he was at school, feeling well and trying to catch up.[7]

As well, dactinomycin can increase the toxic effect of lung radiation by 30 per cent, and reduce the radiation tolerance of the lung by 20 per cent.[8]

Vincristine

Vincristine can cause peripheral neuropathy, which is numbness in your fingers and toes. It comes on gradually and gets worse as your child continues treatment. It usually, although not always, fades away gradually after treatment stops.

You should discuss with the doctor what to do if your child gets peripheral neuropathy. Should the treatment continue and risk permanent damage to the nerves to his or her hands and feet? Or should treatment stop, which brings the risk of missing the benefit of an effective form of chemotherapy?

Vincristine can also cause constipation.

Cyclophosphamide

Cyclophosphamide is a commonly used form of chemotherapy. It can either be taken as a tablet or as an intravenous injection. Its main side effects are:

- bone marrow suppression
- nausea and vomiting
- disturbances of heart rhythm in people with heart disease
- infertility, which is sometimes temporary but can be permanent, especially in men
- baldness (in about 50 per cent of people, usually comes on six weeks after treatment starts)
- metallic taste in the mouth
- blood in the urine.

Blood in the urine is caused by a problem known as haemorrhagic cystitis. It occurs because a chemical produced by the breakdown of the cancer cells is stored in the cells of the bladder. In high enough concentrations, it makes the cells of the bladder bleed.

Your child can avoid this by drinking at least two litres of water every morning before taking the tablets, then another litre or more afterwards. That should flush the chemical out of the bladder.

Bleomycin

Bleomycin is a form of antibiotic used in many types of cancer. It is given either as injections into the muscles or through an intravenous drip.

Bleomycin can cause the usual side effects of baldness, mouth ulcers and fever. It also has a couple of unusual side effects. These are:

- Lung disease known as pulmonary fibrosis; for an unknown reason, occasionally the lungs of people taking bleomycin start to stiffen up, making it hard to breathe. This comes on at least three months after treatment has started, and it is irreversible. It can be fatal. For this reason, if your child is taking bleomycin, he or she will need regular tests to check the lungs are OK.

• Purplish discolouration of the skin creases over joints.
• Odd changes to your child's fingernails.

Methotrexate

Methotrexate can be taken either orally or as intravenous injections. Its main side effects are bone marrow suppression, baldness and damage to the gastrointestinal tract. This shows up as mouth ulcers, or difficulty swallowing, or stomach pains, or diarrhoea, or all of the above. It can also cause:
• skin reactions, especially in the sun
• liver disease
• conjunctivitis
• diarrhoea.
Some of these side effects can be avoided by taking what is known as a folinic acid rescue. If your doctor thinks your child is likely to get these side effects, he or she will prescribe folinic acid. Your child will take the first tablets 24 hours after the dose of methotrexate, then take one tablet every six hours for three or four days. This is very effective at avoiding serious side effects. As well, your child should drink plenty of fluid when taking methotrexate.

Etoposide

Etoposide's main problems are peripheral neuropathy (see vincristine above) and infertility, especially in men. Occasionally, your child can become wheezy and short of breath soon after the injection.

Ifosfamide

Ifosfamide is similar to cyclophosphamide (see above), especially regarding the haemorrhagic cystitis.

Radiotherapy

What is radiotherapy?

Radiotherapy is a treatment for cancer. It uses rays, such as X-rays, gamma rays or electrons, to either cure or control the cancer. The word comes from 'radio', meaning rays, and 'therapy', meaning treatment. It is also known as radiation treatment. It is given by a radiotherapist (also known as a radiation oncologist), who is a doctor specialising in radiotherapy. It works because the rays stop the cancer cells from growing.

Unfortunately, the rays can not tell the difference between the cancer cells and the normal cells in your body. Because cancer cells grow faster than normal cells, they are affected more by radiotherapy. But normal cells are affected, which is the reason side effects occur.

Radiotherapy does not hurt. And it does not make your child radioactive.

Will it cure my child?

Although radiotherapy occasionally cured Ewing's sarcoma in the days before chemotherapy, that was rare. Often the cancer went away, but far more often it came back. Radiotherapy is good at getting rid of the primary tumour—irradiation of a primary limb tumour will get rid of the cancer in about 85 per cent of cases[1]—but evidence suggests it does little to change the chances of survival. It appears to do little to stop metastases. Despite this, radiotherapy increases the chances of survival if given in combination with chemotherapy.

Radiotherapy can also help control Ewing's by stopping it growing or by shrinking it. This can give a longer life, or can help reduce any problems the cancer is giving your child, or both.

Does radiotherapy cause cancer?

Some people who have radiotherapy may later get another form of cancer. However, it is more likely that your treatment will either cure you, or control your cancer. If you are worried about this, talk about it with your radiotherapist.

For more details, see page 314.

How long will the treatment last?

Most people have treatment once a day from Monday to Friday, with a rest on the weekend. A course of treatment usually lasts between two and six weeks. But you should ask your doctor—every person is different.

It is done in a radiotherapy centre which may be attached to the hospital you attend, may be attached to a different hospital or may be in a building on its own.

Each treatment lasts only a few minutes, but you should allow at least an hour at the radiotherapy centre each day. You may have to wait in the waiting room, your child may need blood tests or other X-rays, or you may spend time talking to the radiographer. Once a week, you will talk to the radiotherapist.

Will my child have to stay in hospital?

As long as your child is well enough to be at home, there is no need to be in hospital if radiotherapy is the only treatment. But if your child is sick and in hospital, radiotherapy can be arranged from there. If you live a long way away from the hospital, you may be able to stay in a special hostel or hospital accommodation near the radiotherapy centre. If you need help with transport to the hospital or hostel accommodation, ask your doctor, nurse or social worker what they can arrange.

Exactly how will my child be given the treatment?

Before your child gets radiotherapy, the specialists have to plan how to give it. They work out how to make the machine give the right amount of radiotherapy with the least possible damage to normal cells. This planning can take some time and may mean a few visits to different sections of the hospital for X-rays and scans, as well as the radiotherapy centre.

In the radiotherapy centre, you might have to go to the 'mould room'. Here special moulds can be made to keep parts of your child's body still during treatment. Also, the radiographers will almost certainly use a machine called a 'simulator' to help plan the treatment accurately.

Between them, the radiographers and specialists then use the information from the simulator and any X-rays or scans to work out the dose of rays to give. And they work out exactly where the rays should be directed. This is called the 'treatment field'.

The radiographers are then likely to mark your child's skin so they know where to direct the machine. These marks must not be washed off until the entire treatment is finished. When all this planning has been done, treatment can start.

Each time you go for treatment, the radiographers position your child carefully on the table under the radiotherapy machine. The machine looks very like the simulator where they planned the treatment. Again, your child will feel nothing from this machine.

The radiographers add any moulds they have made, and if necessary they add special shields to protect delicate parts of your child's body.

Then the radiographer leaves the room while the machine is turned on for a few minutes. The radiographers work the machine from a room next door and can see in all the time, either through a window or on a television screen. Your child can speak to them through a microphone or intercom system.

Your child must keep very still when they switch the machine on. It may make a noise and it might move around. It only lasts a few minutes, then that's it.

As treatments go on, your specialists will check how your child is doing. You will probably see the radiotherapist at least once a week, and your child will probably have occasional tests such as scans, blood tests and X-rays.

Is there anything special we should do during treatment?

Yes. There are a few important things to remember:

- Don't wash the marks that the radiographers made. The marks are very important, as they tell them where to direct the rays.
- Don't wash the area that is being treated unless the doctor says it's OK.
- Don't use any ointments, creams, lotions, deodorants, toner, make-up or talcum powder on the treated area, unless the doctor says it's OK.
- Use an electric shaver if you want to shave the treated area—don't use a blade.
- Wear comfortable, loose clothing such as cotton that is not rough on the treated area.
- Keep the treated area out of the sun altogether. It will burn easily.
- Tell your specialist or radiographer about any unusual, painful or worrying problems or side effects. He or she can then make sure that everything is OK. If you keep quiet, he or she won't necessarily know that anything is wrong.
- Eat as well as you can.

How will I know if my child's treatment is working?

Often you won't be able to tell if the treatment is working or not. Your child may well feel worse before feeling better. It is not possible to tell by watching side effects. However, your specialist will watch your child's side effects to check he or she can cope with the amount of radiotherapy being given.

Your radiotherapist can sometimes tell if the treatment is working or not. He or she can do this by doing tests—

X-rays, scans and so on. But it is possible the tests won't show much useful change until some time after the treatment is finished, because there is often a delayed reaction to radiotherapy. In other words, the cancer may not start getting smaller for a while.

Ask your radiotherapist when he or she expects the treatment to start giving results.

Temporary side effects

Some people have no side effects at all during radiotherapy. Others have a few. It depends on what dose of radiotherapy you have and where you have it. There are some side effects that anybody having radiotherapy can get, no matter where the treatment is given. These include:
• feeling tired
• feeling sick
• not wanting to eat
• feeling depressed, down or nervous.
Other side effects occur only if a particular part of the body is being treated. They include:
• red, tanned or itchy skin
• sore or dry mouth or throat
• blocked ears
• losing hair or going bald
• dry cough or feeling short of breath
• having trouble swallowing food
• stomach ache or diarrhoea
• weak bladder.

Feeling tired

Your child may feel very tired. Sometimes this lasts a few weeks after the treatment has ended. It can be because of the treatment itself, or the cancer, or because of the travelling each day.

If this happens, encourage your child to take things easier. Do less than normal. Try doing easier, quieter things. Only do what he or she feels comfortable doing. Rest often.

Feeling sick or vomiting

Many people have radiotherapy without feeling sick at all, but for others it is a problem. It might not start as soon as radiotherapy begins, and it might not go away as soon as radiotherapy finishes.

See pages 312–13 for details on what to do.

Not wanting to eat

Some people have no problems with their appetite during treatment. Others find they don't feel like eating. Or they find their sense of taste changes. This can be because of the treatment, their cancer or just because of the whole experience of having cancer and being treated for it.

It is best for your child to try to eat as well as possible during treatment to maintain strength. If your child doesn't feel like eating, try different foods until you find foods he or she wants to eat. Give smaller amounts more often. Or try special liquid foods which you can get from your pharmacist.

Most cancer councils have booklets and information you might find helpful. Or the hospital may have its own diet information for cancer patients. You can also talk to the hospital dietitian for advice.

Losing hair or going bald

Any hair that is in the way of the rays will come out. This means your child may lose just a patch of head hair or may lose all of it. Radiotherapy to the groin may make his or her pubic hair fall out.

Hair usually starts falling out two or three weeks into the treatment. Your child's scalp may feel hot or itchy just before it starts to fall out.

If your child does lose hair, it will usually grow back again when treatment stops. It takes between four and twelve months to grow back a full head of hair. It may not be as thick as it was before. It can be a slightly different colour. Or it may be finer or curlier than it was before. It can be quite itchy when it's growing back. Frequent shampooing can help the itching. Occasionally after chemotherapy, the hair doesn't grow back properly. Instead it grows back patchily.

Many people find losing their head hair very upsetting. Others don't. Try to remember that it will almost certainly grow back again.

Until it does grow back, your child has a few options. He or she can wear a wig to cover up baldness or patchiness. If this suits, it is a good idea to get a wig fitted before your child starts losing hair, so it is ready when it does fall out. Also, this makes it easier to match the colour.

Many hospitals have a wig bank or library. You may be able to borrow a free wig from them. Or if you are on a low income you may be able to get a free wig under special government schemes. Some support groups have wig banks or libraries too. If you want to buy one, expect to pay between $100 and $600 for a synthetic one, and around $1000 for one made out of real hair. And note that wigs made of real hair can take more time and money to look after than synthetic ones. If you are in a private health fund, you may be able to get some of this cost back (but check with the fund before you buy). Ask your doctor, nurse or the hospital social worker for more information about how to go about getting free wigs or where to buy them.

Some people don't bother with a wig—they stay bald, or cover up with a scarf or hat. A bald head can be a fashion statement, especially for a child or teenager who would like to look a bit different. It's up to your child. There is no medical reason why a wig is necessary, and it is far better to be happy and bald than self-conscious about a wig.

The only thing about going bald is that your child's scalp will be more sensitive to the sun than usual. He or she should wear a hat or a high protection suncream (SPF 15+) when in the sun.

Sore or dry mouth or throat

Being treated on the head or neck may give you a sore mouth or mouth ulcers. This is because the cells that make up the lining of your mouth can be affected by the rays.

It is wise to keep teeth, gums and mouth very clean during treatment, to help stop infections. The nurses can show you how to do this. Your child should use a very soft toothbrush or a cotton bud for teeth and gums, or brush his or her teeth with fingers, rather than a toothbrush.

Your specialists may supply a special liquid mouthwash to use for a red or sore mouth. You can make one yourself by mixing 1 teaspoon of salt, 1 teaspoon of baking soda (sodium bicarbonate) in 1200 ml of warm water. Use it three times a day after meals. Don't use a commercial mouthwash.

Your child should eat soft foods and drink plenty of fluids, but not anything with a high acid level such as grapefruit, tomato or orange. Spicy foods and any particular food or drink that stings should be avoided. If it does, don't eat it. A lip salve or ointment on your lips can help stop them drying out.

If your child is having trouble swallowing because of a sore and dry mouth or throat, try some of these ideas:
• suck on ice blocks
• drink lots of liquids
• moisten foods with butter
• dunk biscuits in tea
• blend foods
• eat soups and ice creams
• ask your dentist, doctor or nurse about artificial saliva
• avoid cigarette smoke.

Itchy skin and other skin problems

Your child's skin may go red and itchy or may appear tanned where the rays go through. This is only likely to happen if a part of the body near the skin's surface is being treated. It usually happens only towards the end of treatment.

It will clear up soon after treatment ends, but the skin may feel a bit stretched or thinner in that area forever. And your child may lose some of the hairs on that part of the skin permanently.

It is a good idea to always either cover up that piece of skin, or use a high protection suncream (SPF 15+). It will probably be much more sensitive to the sun than it was before.

If the radiographers marked your child's skin, make sure the mark stays there. If the radiotherapist says so, you may be able to splash the area that's being treated with warm water. Then pat it gently dry. Don't use any soap, make-up, perfume, deodorant, ointment, lotion or cream on that part—they can make the skin even more sore. Don't put on any tight or rough clothes.

Keep the skin from becoming too hot or too cold. So

don't use a hot water bottle. You can heat the bed with an electric blanket, but turn it off before your child gets into bed. Don't use a heat lamp. Don't use a cold cloth or ice-pack. Keep the skin covered if it's either cold or hot outside. Keep it away from sunlight.

Tell your doctor or nurse if it hurts too much. They may be able to help.

Stomach aches or diarrhoea

This may happen if your child is having radiotherapy to the stomach, back or groin. Ask your doctor if he or she can have something to help if the aches get too bad. Try the following suggestions to ease diarrhoea:
- eat warm or cold rather than hot foods
- add low fibre foods such as bananas or macaroni to the diet
- don't eat high fibre foods like raw fruits, vegetables and bread
- drink lots of liquid to replace the fluid you are losing
- eat smaller amounts of food more often
- don't eat foods like cabbage, fizzy drinks, highly spiced food or beans that can cause cramp
- don't eat dairy foods like milk or cheese.
If it lasts longer than 24 hours, tell your doctor.

Feeling depressed, down or nervous

Some people find the treatment difficult to deal with. It can seem to go on forever. It can be difficult to know whether your child is getting better or worse. If this is what is worrying you, ask your specialist how things are going.

Going for the treatment may make your child, or anyone else in your family, depressed or nervous. There is no right or wrong way to feel. But it is always best to try and be as hopeful and positive as possible. Remember that many people are alive and well years after finishing their radiotherapy treatment.

It is a good idea to talk to your child about his or her feelings whenever possible. Many children feel their parents are not honest with them, and are scared that something else is going on that they do not know about. Remember that you do not have cancer—your child does.

You should also talk about your own feelings to your child, your partner, family or friends. Talking often helps. If you don't feel like talking with people who are close to you, you can talk to the hospital social worker or nurse. Or you may want to talk to people who have been through the same sort of experience as you. Ask your nurse or hospital social worker about how to get in touch with someone who has been through the same sort of experience.

Blocked ears

Radiotherapy to your child's head can make his or her ears blocked. If this happens, tell your radiographer or specialist—don't try and clear them yourself.

Dry cough or feeling short of breath

This may happen if your child is having radiotherapy to the chest. If so, tell your specialist or nurse immediately. They may be able to help.

Weak bladder

If your child is having treatment near the bladder, he or she might complain of needing to pass urine more often. This should go back to normal when treatment ends.

Permanent side effects

Your child could have some permanent side effects, depending on exactly when and where the radiotherapy was given.

Attempts are being made to reduce the incidence of permanent side effects by using hyperfractionated therapy, in which two smaller doses are given each day rather than one large one. The belief is that this can allow doctors to use a higher dose overall but with fewer side effects.[2] Permanent problems, depending on the site of irradiation, can include:

- curvature of the spine, which can come on two years after radiotherapy to the ribs

- failure of development of a breast
- chronic cystitis, particularly if patient had cyclophosphamideas part of chemotherapy
- death of the bone at the top of the femur, or thighbone
- stiffening of joints
- shortening of limb
- liver and kidney damage.

Other problems include the risk of developing a second cancer. See page 315 for details. One of the most important risks is that of damage to bones.

Damaged bones

The effect of radiation on bones has been known since the turn of the century, when one researcher irradiated day-old chicks and found their growth was stunted. And they have been known about in children since 1930.

This problem is decreasing for three reasons:
- other forms of therapy have improved so much that sometimes radiation can be eliminated from the treatment without reducing the chances of success;
- better education has meant that patients and their

families are better prepared to deal with problems that arise; and

• prostheses and surgery have been developed which offer previously handicapped people a better chance of a normal life.

For all these reasons, doctors prefer to avoid using radiotherapy in younger children.

The most obvious place that irradiation damages bone growth is at the growth plate, located at the ends of bones. If these are damaged, then bone growth can slow down or even stop. But every other part of the bone—including the marrow, the blood supply and the cartilage—can be damaged by radiotherapy.

If the main part of the bone is damaged, the result can be that calcium is not absorbed properly, so the bones weaken and bend. All the different types of damage together make irradiated bone susceptible to fracture.

Radiation can affect every bone in the body—long bones like the thigh bone, flat bones like the skull, joints and even teeth.[3] Radiation to the spine can produce scoliosis, which means curvature of the spine. Radiation to a child's face can cause severe abormalities if growth of some bones is retarded. These facial deformities are difficult to correct and can cause psychological scars which remain long after cosmetic surgery has repaired the physical damage.

Irradiated joints become arthritic. Eventually, the joint may become quite difficult to move and movement in some directions might be lost altogether.

The teeth are extraordinarily sensitive to radiation. Even small doses can stop second teeth from coming down, and moderate doses can cause poor alignment of the jaws and cavities in teeth.

Measures which help prevention of and recovery from damage include:

• rehabilitation during and after radiotherapy to prevent joint stiffness and work around abnormalities;

Length and predicted growth of femur (centimetres) in boys and girls

Age (years)	Mean length	Expected total growth	Growth from proximal epiphysis	Growth from distal epiphysis
Boys				
6	28	19	6	13
8	32	15	4.5	10.5
10	36	11	3.5	7.5
12	40	7	2	5
14	44	3	1	2
16	46	0.5	0	0.5
Girls				
6	28	15	4.5	10.5
8	33	11	4	7
10	37	7	2.5	4.5
12	41	3	1	2
14	43	0.5	0.5	0
16	44	0	0	0

Length and predicted growth of tibia (centimetres)

Age (years)	Mean length	Expected total growth	Growth from proximal epiphysis	Growth from distal epiphysis
Boys				
6	22	15	9	6
8	25	12	7	5
10	29	9	5	4
12	32	5	3	2
14	35	2	1.5	0.5
16	37	0	0	0
Girls				
6	23	12	7	5
8	26	9	5	4
10	29	6	3.5	2.5
12	33	2	1	1
14	34	0.5	0.5	0
16	35	0	0	0

Source: Anderson M., Green W. T. & Messner M. D. Growth and prediction of growth in the lower extremities. *Journal of Bone and Joint Surgery* 1963; **45**: 1–14.

- prostheses to correct limb length abnormalities;
- reconstructive surgery where profound abnormalities exist;
- high pressure oxygen if necrosis to the jaw-bone is considered a possibility.

Radiotherapy is now designed to exclude the far end of any long bone involved, so that end keeps growing. This should partly ease the problem of stunted growth. For example, irradiating the femur of a 6-year-old boy could lead to a loss of growth of 19 cm (see table). But if you can spare the growth plate at the bottom of the femur, near the knee, then you would lose only 6 cm of growth. While still a significant loss of growth, that makes the difference between a possible amputation and a built-up heel.

Radiotherapy is also designed to miss a corridor of bone down the limb. This is to prevent an occasional complication in which the soft tissue around the irradiated bone contracts as it become fibrous. If this goes all the way around the bone it could constrict the blood flow down the bone, causing part of it to die.

A group of American orthopaedic surgeons decided to follow up every child who had been treated with radiotherapy for childhood cancer and who survived to the stage where their bones stop growing—the age of 14 for girls and 16 for boys.[4] They found 143 people who fitted the criteria.

Fifty of them had developed scoliosis—that is, a sideways curvature of the spine. Only three out of those 50 needed treatment with a brace to try to straighten the back, while the rest were expected to get straighter with time. A further fourteen developed kyphosis, or a hunch back. While looking unusual, only one of those fourteen had surgery to try correct the problem.

As well, twelve developed a shortened leg with the difference between the two legs ranging from 2 cm to 9 cm. Some had no treatment, some wore built up shoes while four of them had an operation. Seven girls had one smaller breast on the side that received radiotherapy; 51 had deformities of the ribs or chest; 23 complained of chronic pain at or near the tumour site. Three patients developed a second cancer.

Experts say that while these long-term effects are undoubtedly serious, they are less common than they used to be.

Surgery

The role of surgery is changing. Years ago, it was thought useless to operate on Ewing's sarcoma because of the high chance that it had already spread. What's the point of an operation if the cancer is just going to appear somewhere else?

But because of the advances in chemotherapy, it is now more feasible to operate. An operation that gets rid of the primary tumour, combined with intensive chemo-therapy, can now give hopes of a cure in many people with Ewing's sarcoma.

It has also been recognised that using radiotherapy alone to get rid of the primary tumour can cause severe long-term damage to a limb. Surgery may provide a more predictable and reparable form of damage.

Surgeons used to try to remove just the tumour and little else. But now more extensive operations are in vogue for a number of reasons. First, too many people had their tumours return at the operation site when only small amounts of tissue around the tumour were removed. Second, artificial limbs, known as prostheses, have improved considerably and the loss of a limb no longer restricts mobility as it once did. Third, surgeons have developed 'limb-sparing' techniques in which plenty of tissue can be removed around the tumour, to give as big a margin of safety as possible, but the arm or leg can be made useful again through the clever use of existing muscles and bones.

Doctors also recognised that in a child younger than six or eight with a cancer in the leg, radiotherapy is likely to cause a drastically shortened limb. It may be better to amputate at the knee, and fit a prosthesis, than have one leg 25 cm or more shorter than the other.[1] Usually, it is possible to compensate for a leg shortened by 6–8 cm with a built up shoe. Any more shortening and a special prosthesis is usually needed.[2]

Many bones in the body, believe it or not, are quite expendable. People can get by perfectly well without many bones of the hands and feet, the collarbone and the shoulder blade. Often if the tumour is in these bones, doctors recommend removal of the entire bone. This can also be done for small tumours of the ribs, the fibula (the outer, thinner bone on the lower leg), parts of the spine and parts of the pelvis.[3]

Will surgery help?

The answer to this is not definite, but it looks as though surgery does help in many cases. In theory, surgery should help. The aim is to reduce the risk of the primary tumour coming back, which should improve the chances of survival. But against that, having surgery may delay beginning chemotherapy, particularly if the wound becomes infected, and an operation is a large stress on a body already under strain.

The trend is towards operating on small tumours that look easy to remove, such as those in the rib, the hand, the foot and occasionally in the pelvis. While doctors expect these operations to improve survival, there have not yet been any good long-term studies to check this out.

What types of operations are there?

There are as many different operations, and variations on those different operations, as there are surgeons. Many different factors influence what type of operation is needed. These include:
- size of the tumour
- exactly where it is
- whether it is in bone or soft tissue
- whether it has spread from its primary site into surrounding tissues
- whether it has spread to distant organs such as the lungs
- general health of the person with the tumour
- age and usual physical activity level of the person with the tumour.[4]

The aim of every operation is to remove as much as possible of the cancer and disturb as little as possible of the surrounding tissue. On top of that, surgeons aim to make sure they have a taken out a margin of apparently normal tissue around the cancer. This is so that if any of it has spread beyond what looks like the margin of the tumour, then the chances are higher that it has been removed, too. Ideally, this margin should be 10 cm.

But to fit those criteria, anything can happen. For a small sarcoma in the little finger that doesn't seem to have spread, the finger would probably be removed. A large tumour of the foot that seems to be spreading up to the ankle might cause an amputation of the foot. Somebody with a 15 cm sarcoma of the pelvis might have a short course of chemotherapy with or without radiotherapy followed by surgery to 'debulk' the tumour—that is, get rid of most of it. That gives the following chemotherapy and radiotherapy a better chance to work.

Every case is worked out differently. Part of the reason for that is that few surgeons see enough people with Ewing's sarcoma to really develop that special knowledge that surgeons operating on more common diseases such as breast cancer or bowel cancer can get. So they do what they think is best and compare their results with those of doctors in other nations. In the end surgeons learn which types of operation are more effective than others, but it is a much slower process for Ewing's sarcoma than it is for more common tumours.

So for tumours of the limbs there are two choices—amputation or limb-sparing surgery, in which every attempt is made to preserve the arm or leg as intact as possible.

Amputation

Sometimes amputation is thought to be the best option. This is the case if an operation to remove only the tumour would leave an arm or leg that didn't work properly. Amputation is better when prostheses—artificial limbs—work well, such as those fitted for amputations below the knee.

In most cases, artificial limbs can be fitted. Prostheses for lower limbs are generally better and more effective than prostheses for upper limbs, although these are improving all the time.

Recovery after amputation and the fitting of a prosthesis is remarkably rapid. After the insertion of a lower limb prosthesis, many people are up and walking in a plaster after a week.

However, pain can be a chronic problem—oddly, pain in the limb that is no longer there. This is known as 'phantom pain' or a 'phantom limb'. The person feels like the affected arm or leg is still there, and still hurts.

Even though the limb is not there, painkillers seem to work.

Limb-sparing surgery

The alternative operation—the limb-sparing operation—can leave a person with cancer with his or her natural limb. Muscles are turned and adapted, bone grafts can be used. In some operations existing bones are even turned back to front. Anything can be done to make the limb usable. In many cases, prostheses are still needed, although they are different from those used in amputation.

Prostheses are usually inserted at the same time the tumour is removed, although occasionally a temporary one is inserted, to be replaced some months later by a more permanent fixture. They are usually made of either stainless steel or an alloy of the metals chromium, cobalt and molybdenum.

This type of surgery is highly specialised, and needs to be done by an expert. The range of operations available is too great to cover in this book, but your surgeon will be able to give advice on whether a limb-sparing operation is feasible.

A warning. Despite the attractiveness of leaving the limb there (it looks better than an amputation), people who have amputations may find they are more active and mobile than people who have limb-sparing operations. After all, there is nothing to damage or look after, because it is not there.

Surgery to the trunk

Two choices also exist for tumours of the trunk—excision with a wide margin or debulking. In the first type every effort is made to remove the whole tumour and some tissue around it as a margin of safety.

In the second type, surgeons remove as much of the tumour as possible. If this type of surgery is carried out, it is usually done either because the tumour was in too awkward a position to remove it all, or there are signs that the tumour has spread throughout the body and there would be no clear benefit from the extra damage done through removing the whole tumour. Debulking surgery does not imply that there is no hope for a cure— sometimes the aim is to make the tumour small enough so that radiotherapy and chemotherapy are more effective in removing it altogether.

Surgery for lung metastases

The most common site for metastases with Ewing's sarcoma is the lung. Sometimes people with Ewing's have two or three clear metastases in the lung, with no signs of any others. These have proved difficult to treat with chemotherapy alone. But it seems that if the conditions are right, the surgery to remove the metastases can improve survival by enough to make it worth the effects of surgery. Of course, this is done in conjunction with chemotherapy.

It is fairly well recognised that as long as surgery is only undertaken on suitable patients, about 33 per cent will be alive three years after the operation and 25 per cent alive five years after the operation. French surgeons even report that one of nineteen patients who have had operations for lung metastases is alive eleven years later, apparently cured.[5]

In one study from the US National Cancer Institute, of nineteen patients who had operations for lung metastases, six had tumours too large to remove and three had benign lung disease that was unrelated to Ewing's sarcoma. Ten people had their metastases removed. The average survival for those who had metastases removed was 28 months, compared to the twelve months average survival of those whose tumours were too large to remove. At the time this work was reported, three patients were still alive 12, 36 and 61 months after the operation.[6]

It is important that the operation be carried out only on those who have developed lung metastases but still have a fair chance of survival. These people are:

• those who were free of disease for more than a year before the lung metastases appeared
• those with few metastases (say, less than ten)
• those without any other metastases
• those whose general health is good.

Complications of surgery

Infection

Operations involving bone are prone to deep-seated infections. If the infection is in the bone, then this is known as osteomyelitis. This can be a particularly difficult infection to get rid of, requiring weeks in hospital on intravenous antibiotics and months on antibiotic tablets. Sometimes an operation is even required to try to clear out the infection.

It is possible to get post-operative infections that do not involve the bone. These are likely to be called cellulitis, and merely involve an infection of the skin. Cellulitis is easier to treat than osteomyelitis.

Recurrence

Although people who have surgery are less likely to have a recurrence of the sarcoma than those who have radiotherapy without surgery, a recurrence is still possible. The most likely reason for a tumour to come back in the same place after surgery is that the surgeon did not get all of it in the first place.

It is possible to have metastases, or secondary cancers, develop somewhere else in the body long after surgery removed the primary tumour. This occurs because the cancer had spread before surgery, even though it had not shown up. Because of this risk, most people with Ewing's sarcoma now have chemotherapy as the first line of treatment.

Disturbance of function

One of the complications of surgery is a disturbance of function—things do not work as well afterwards. For example, if a nerve is damaged then there may be numbness, or an inability to move certain muscles. These problems may be temporary or they may be permanent. Or if an artery is damaged, the blood supply may be limited, which means the muscles may tire more easily than before the operation. If a bone is removed, then the limb may or may not work as well as before. It is important to discuss *before* any operation exactly what is likely to happen. If you are prepared, you can deal with the consequences of surgery better.

Mechanical problems

In any sort of operation where screws or pins or plates are used, as in many operations involving bones, things can go wrong. Screws can work loose, pins can fall out and plates can break. It is impossible to say how often these things happen because every operation is different. But they do happen.

Pneumonia

There is a slight risk of pneumonia after an operation involving a general anaesthetic. This occurs because the lungs don't inflate as fully as they should during the operation, and because it is hard to breathe as deeply as you should after an operation.

However pneumonia is fairly rare in children and teenagers and young adults after an operation. It is more common in older people and in those who smoke. If a younger person gets pneumonia, it is usually easily treatable with antibiotics.

Death

There is a small risk of death during any operation involving a general anaesthetic. In Australia, that risk is something like 1 in 100,000.

Pain and Other Problems

Pain is one of the biggest problems with cancer. Between 30 per cent and 50 per cent of all people having treatment for cancer and at least three-quarters of all people with advanced cancer have pain.[1,2] It is also one of the problems people fear most when they hear the word cancer. They think the pain is uncontrollable.

The truth is not quite as bad as that. The pain of cancer can be very bad for some people, although some others have little pain from their cancer. The pain of cancer can be hard to control, although many people manage the pain quite easily.

Some doctors will say: 'there is no pain that can't be brought under control'. To some extent that is true—in the right circumstances. But unfortunately not everyone is treated in the ideal circumstances, by the ideal doctors and nurses, in the ideal hospital. Some people do suffer from the pain.

However there is always something that can be done to help control it. There are drugs such as Panadeine Forte, Codral Forte, codeine and morphine. If pain is limited to one region, then there are operations that can be done to interfere with the nerves to that region, so reducing the pain.

It is worth remembering that nobody except the person experiencing the pain can really judge what it is, or how bad it is. In fact, that forms one of the most common definitions of pain.

Pain is whatever the experiencing person says it is and exists whenever he/she says it does.

Children's pain

Little is known about the pain children feel from cancer.[3] In fact, until the 1970s doctors and researchers rarely thought much about the pain children feel from cancer and from its treatment. Those who did think about it thought that children with cancer experienced less pain than adults.[4]

It was not until the early 1980s that doctors really started trying to assess how much pain children with cancer suffered. But even then, they only looked at the small proportion of children who needed specialised care for their pain—they did not consider the whole population of children with cancer.

A group of Canadian psychologists and doctors decided to work out how much pain the average child with cancer suffered. To do this, they asked every child over seven (and the parents of every child under seven) who attended their outpatients clinic to rate the pain on a scale of one to ten. Most of these children had leukaemia, and most of the rest had lymphomas. However the results are relevant to all children with cancer.

About half the children said they had experienced severe pain at some stage from their cancer. About a quarter said they had experienced severe pain at some stage from their chemotherapy. About a sixth said they had experienced severe pain at some stage from having blood taken.

Children also said that lumbar punctures, in which a needle is stuck in the child's back to drain fluid out of the spinal canal for examination, and bone marrow aspirations (see page 248) were very painful.

Several important findings came from this study. One was that generally parents' estimates of pain were fairly close to the children's estimates of pain. Another was that it showed, clearly and unequivocally, that children experience pain from the cancer, from its diagnosis and from its treatment. A third was that it showed that children generally suffer more pain before they are diagnosed with cancer. Once they are diagnosed and treatment starts, the pain usually recedes.

Of course this study did not look at children who are dying of their cancer and whose active treatment has stopped. In many cases, the pain in the final stages of cancer can be worse than it ever was.

The Canadians make the point that it is not good enough to treat pain only when children complain of it. For one thing, many children and parents think pain is inevitable and uncontrollable, so they do not complain. For another, giving painkillers after the pain has become severe is not nearly as effective as giving them before the pain gets to that stage.

A point to remember about pain: the word pain comes from the Greek word 'poine', which means punishment. Younger children sometimes accept their pain and do not complain about it because they think it is punishment for something they have done wrong. Always ask about pain.

Types of pain

Four main types of pain exist. These are:

- Bone pain—due to either the primary or secondary cancers, this pain is usually felt deep inside and is well localised to the site of the tumour. It is often worse at night.
- Visceral pain—this is due to cancer in one of the viscera, or internal organs. It can be either a constant or a colicky intermittent type of ache, and it can often be hard to pin down to just one spot.
- Neuropathic pain—this is due to the cancer affecting the nerves. It is often a burning pain, and the area that is painful might feel super-sensitive to the touch.
- Pain due to cancer treatment, whether it be surgery, chemotherapy or radiotherapy.

As well as these, pain can be either acute (sudden, recent onset) or chronic (going for a long time).

It is possible, particularly if cancer has spread, to have different types of pain in different parts of the body. For example, you could have bone pain in the back, visceral pain under the ribs and neuropathic pain in the leg. Knowing what causes the pain can often help the treatment of it. This can be particularly important if the pain is neuropathic, because sometimes narcotic drugs, such as codeine and morphine, which are the ones most commonly used against cancer pain, do not work against neuropathic pain.

Painkilling drugs

Narcotics

The two most commonly used drugs are codeine and morphine. These are both narcotic drugs; they belong to the same class of drugs as illegal narcotics such as heroin.

For that reason, there has long been a prejudice against using morphine.

But recently the prejudice against morphine has started to ease, and doctors are now realising that it is a very safe and effective drug against the severe pain of cancer. It is available as a syrup and as long-acting tablets, so injections are no longer necessary except in certain circumstances. And it works.

When a person with cancer starts morphine, the dose needed quickly increases. That is because the body adapts very quickly to lowish doses of morphine. The dose may even need to be increased every two to three days for the first week or two. But eventually a point will be reached where the morphine is doing its job, and it will stay effective for a longer period. Eventually, though, the dose will have to be increased again. People who start taking 5 mg of morphine every four hours may end up taking 1000 mg every four hours—a dose that would kill someone who has never taken morphine before. But the body adapts to the morphine so effectively that these enormous doses are both safe and what is needed.

The main problem with morphine is that it causes drowsiness and sedation and, in large doses, can cause confusion. Just as the body adapts to morphine and the doses need to relieve pain must be increased, so does the body adapt to the sedative effect of morphine. Doses that would put you or I to sleep immediately are swallowed eagerly by a two-year-old who has become used to it.

Morphine also causes constipation. This can be a problem if you already have advanced cancer and are not getting a lot of exercise or eating a good diet. For that reason, most doctors recommend that anybody taking morphine regularly should also be taking laxatives every day.

Another problem with morphine is that it can make the person taking it sick. Nausea and vomiting can be quite severe at first. But they usually settle down within a week, although every time the dose is increased some nausea may return. Sometimes it is a good idea to start taking drugs against nausea, such as Maxolon or Stemetil, whenever morphine is started or the dose increased.

Other, rarer, problems exist. Morphine can make the person taking it itchy, for no known reason. It can also occasionally cause blood vessels in the eye to burst—this looks bad but is quite harmless and repairs itself within a couple of weeks.

Morphine tablets are now available which last for twelve hours, meaning medication does not have to be given nearly as often. These are very good for people who can take tablets but if they can't, the syrup is still available.

There is no limit to the amount of morphine you can take, as long as the dose is increased gradually. If pain increases, then the dose should be increased to the point where either relief is felt or intolerable side effects occur.

Codeine is a similar drug to morphine, in that it can cause constipation and drowsiness. It is very good against mild to moderate pain, especially in combination with aspirin or paracetamol. It is not strong enough to use on severe pain.

Oxycodone is another narcotic which is somewhat similar to codeine. It works more quickly, although the benefit may not last as long.

There is a myth that people who take morphine automatically become addicted. It is untrue. Many people take morphine for a while when they need it, then stop taking it when the pain eases. Addiction to morphine is not at all common.

Anti-inflammatories

Sometimes drugs more commonly used against arthritis, such as Indocid, Naprosyn, Brufen or Dolobid, are used to ease the pain of cancer. These are known as non-steroidal anti-inflammatory drugs, or NSAIDs.

Most of the time, they are given in conjunction with morphine and they make the morphine work better. Sometimes they are used as the first treatment for pain. If they are not effective, then you can move up to codeine or morphine.

Usually, if these drugs are going to work they will do so within a week or so. If they are not effective, then it is best to either switch to another drug in the class or to drop them altogether.[2]

Antidepressants

Often antidepressants are prescribed for neuropathic pain. There are two reasons for this—one is that sometimes they work and the second is that often not much else does.

Antiepileptic drugs

These, too, are sometimes used to treat sharp, stabbing neuropathic pain. Sometimes they work, sometimes they don't.[2]

Steroid hormones

If used for a short period, while waiting for other drugs like morphine to take effect and reach the best dose, steroids such as prednisone can be very good for severe pain.[2]

Other methods

Radiotherapy

A short course of radiotherapy can be an extremely effective way of controlling localised pain, especially if it is coming from a bone. It can shrink the tumour enough so that it stops causing the pressure that is causing the pain. See page 277–93 for more details.

Chemotherapy

If a tumour responds to chemotherapy, it will shrink. That will cause pain to ease. See pages 257–76 for more details.

Local anaesthetics and surgery

Doctors have tried a variety of methods to relieve pain that has not been eased by the usual methods. They can inject local anaesthetic into and around the spinal cord, or around particular nerves. They can even operate to cut particular nerves. Sometimes these methods work brilliantly, sometimes they do little good.[1]

Marijuana

Marijuana is good at relieving both the stress and the pain of cancer. It doesn't do the job on its own—it should be used in conjunction with other legal drugs. The fact that marijuana is illegal makes it difficult to use.

Heroin

Every now and then a story appears in the newspapers that heroin should be allowed to be used for people with cancer. It is true that heroin is effective, but it is no more effective than morphine. There really is no need for it; morphine does everything that heroin can do, except give that addictive 'rush' when first injected.

Drugs by other means

There are a whole host of ways that painkilling drugs can be given, if tablets or syrups are too hard to take. They can be given by suppository, through continuous infusions into the skin or through continuous intravenous infusions. In situations where the pain is almost impossible to relieve and the person is confined to bed, painkillers can be given directly into the fluid surrounding the spinal cord through a semi-permanent epidural line.[2]

These methods are all slightly more difficult to use than swallowing tablets or syrups. Having infusions going is definitely a bother, and usually (but not always) means a stay in hospital. But they work.

Other problems

Weight loss

Many people with advanced cancer lose a lot of weight. This is partly because they are so sick they lose their appetite, and partly because the cancer consumes so much of the body's energy.

It would be good to be able to improve the appetite of people with advanced cancer, as getting them to put on weight makes them stronger and less susceptible to infections and other illnesses. Unfortunately, most attempts to do so have not been too successful.

There are a number of drugs that can be used to stimulate appetite.[1] These include:
• Maxolon (a drug used to control nausea and vomiting)
• prednisolone (a steroid hormone)
• Cyproheptadine
• progesterone.
Various other ideas have been tried. One was to give a

drip containing plenty of calories. While this seems a fine idea, it doesn't seem to do any good in most cases.

Weakness

Although weakness is a common symptom of advanced cancer, doctors understand little about why it happens. Because so little is known about why it happens, little can be done to treat it.

Some trials have been done which show that steroid hormones can improve the strength and mobility of people with advanced cancer. This improvement starts only two to three days after starting the drugs. However the effect seems to be fairly short-lived, perhaps lasting as little as three weeks or so.[1]

It is early days for research, but it is possible that some amphetamines might help make some people with advanced cancer less weak.

Nausea and vomiting

Nausea and vomiting are common in people who have cancer. It might be due to a physical problem of the cancer, such as that it involves the stomach, or the mere presence of a cancer in the body making your child feel sick.

Nausea and vomiting are also common in people having radiotherapy and, in particular, chemotherapy.

If your child feels sick, try any of the ideas below. They might help. Your child should:
- Eat lightly before each treatment if the sickness comes before treatments.
- Don't eat for a few hours before each treatment if the sickness comes straight after treatments.
- Eat smaller amounts more often.
- Eat slowly and chew well to help digest your food better.
- Do not drink during mealtimes.

- Try not to eat sweet or fatty things.
- Eat dry toast or dry biscuits—they often help.
- Drink clear, cool and unsweetened drinks like apple juice.
- Avoid anything too strenuous after a meal, but try not to lie down for at least two hours after a meal.
- Learn relaxation or meditation methods.

As well, medication exists which can help. The traditional drugs used are Stemetil (chemical name prochlorperazine) and Maxolon (chemical name metaclopramide). These drugs can have significant side effects, and are generally not used in children unless needed, although they are safer in teenagers and young adults. They can be effective.

A more effective drug released on the Australian market in 1992 is Ondansetron. It is very expensive and only available through some hospitals. At the time of writing, not every child with cancer would be guaranteed to have Ondansetron, even if it was needed.

Later Physical Effects of Cancer and its Treatment

Obviously it's a worry—what happens later? Does having had cancer once make it likely a second one will happen? Or does it mean that somehow you are protected from a second one? All that surgery and chemotherapy and radiotherapy must have some impact on the body—will my child be infertile? Or somehow different?

These questions are becoming a worry for more and more people, because childhood cancer is fairly common. By the age of twenty, one in every 1000 people has been cured of cancer.[1] And a survey done at the Children's Hospital of Philadelphia, which has one of the largest and longest running clinics for survivors of childhood cancer, found that 73 per cent of patients coming to the clinic had some residual affect of the cancer or its treatment and 41 per cent were severely affected.[1]

Second cancers

It has long been known that radiation could cause cancer. Bone sarcomas were noted among workers who painted radium on watch dials to make them glow as far back as 1929. The link between therapeutic irradiation and bone sarcomas was established in 1948, but even today not enough is known about the problem.

For example, it was common practice after World War II to treat children with ringworm of the scalp with radiation therapy. It worked, but they proved later in life to be susceptible to cancer, especially cancers of the bones.

Some people who have radiation for Ewing's sarcoma develop a second bone cancer some years later. The most common second cancer seen is osteosarcoma, rather than Ewing's sarcoma.[2] Others include lymphomas and thyroid cancer.[3]

Genetics may play a part, because second tumours have occurred outside the radiation field. If it was purely due to the radiation, then all tumours would occur in bone that had been irradiated.

As well, there have been cases of acute leukaemia developing after therapy, as well as one case which appeared between the time of diagnosis and treatment

Younger children appear more likely to develop a second cancer than older children.

But how many is some? That is hard to say. A group of twenty doctors from the USA, France, Italy, England, the Netherlands and Canada have formed the Late Effects Study Group, which aims to look at the long-term impact of chemotherapy and radiotherapy.

In one study they followed up more than 9000 children who had survived cancer for at least two years. They found that these children who had been treated for cancer were 133 times more likely to develop a bone cancer than children who had never had cancer. In other words, treatment for a first cancer greatly increases the risk of a second cancer.[4]

In particular, the risk of a second bone cancer was increased by more than 600 times if the child's original tumour was a Ewing's sarcoma. There was a 22 per cent chance that a child successfully treated for Ewing's sarcoma would develop a second bone cancer within twenty years.

Two factors were particularly important—the type of chemotherapy used and the dose of radiotherapy used.

The type of chemotherapy most closely associated with a second cancer was the use of alkylating agents. This is a class of drugs that includes cyclophosphamide, chlorambucil and triethylenemelamine (now rarely used).

The dose of radiotherapy was important. Children at highest risk of developing a second cancer were those who received more than 6000 rads (a rad is a measurement of radiation). While it is difficult to describe how much a rad is, a radiotherapist would be able to describe, for any given course of treatment, how many rads he or she is planning to give. A dose of 6000 rads is fairly high, but it is not unusual for a child to be given that dose. Unfortunately, doses of 5000 to 6000 rads are those recommended as giving the best chance of getting rid of the primary tumour.[5]

The site of the second bone cancers was unusual—34 per cent occurred in the jaw or skull, 38 per cent in the skeleton and 28 per cent in the long bones of the arms and legs. This compares to the usual distribution of primary bone cancers of 4 per cent, 21 per cent and 72 per cent respectively.

Another factor that was found to be important was that younger children were more likely to develop a second cancer than older children.

But the figures from the Late Effects Study Group were unusually high. Doctors from the Istituto Ortopedico

Rizzoli in Bologna, Italy, examined the records of all 255 people treated at the institute for Ewing's sarcoma between 1950 and 1982.[6] They found that 78 patients were at risk of developing a tumour—that is, they had been treated with radiotherapy and had survived more than three years.

Only three of these people developed a second cancer at the site of the irradiation—two have apparently been cured by treatment. Interestingly, all three who had gone through chemotherapy for their first tumour refused it for the second. All three had been treated with doses higher than 6000 rads. They suggest the chance of second tumours is a factor in favour of surgery.

But a study from California suggests the risks are much more modest—only two out of 25 who had survived Ewing's developed a second cancer.[7]

There has also been a report that the chances of developing a second cancer, usually osteosarcoma, after treatment for Ewing's sarcoma is about 35 per cent by the time ten years have passed.[8]

It is possible that the risk of a second cancer will decline among those people treated now with radiotherapy.
Until the early 1970s, the type of radiotherapy used was called orthovoltage. This was absorbed strongly by bone. But now radiotherapists use megavoltage, which allows the rays to be absorbed more evenly and not concentrate in the bone. This might mean that the chances of developing a second bone tumour will decrease in the future.[7]

Will my child be infertile?

Cancer and infertility are more alike than you realise. Those who are infertile and those with cancer both feel sad about lost potential, and both are supremely sensitive to the passage of time. Both feel their bodies are failing to function properly, and both feel a sense of injured self-esteem. Both ask 'why me?' Both have to ward off depression and maintain hope. Both will submit to almost any treatment, no matter how painful or humiliating, in the hope of achieving their goal.[9]

The infertility that might result from cancer treatment is often handled poorly. When a young person is diagnosed with cancer, the most important thing seems to be starting treatment. Other issues such as infertility are pushed into the background. But assuming this young person survives the cancer, as half or more do, then that person is going to have to deal with issues raised by the cancer for the rest of his or her life. At the time of diagnosis, and throughout treatment, the person with cancer and his or her family need accurate information about infertility.

But accurate information is not easy to find. The best information on fertility comes from an enormous study of more than 2000 people in the United States who had survived having cancer as a child or teenager. It took two and a half years for researchers to carry out one-hour interviews with all the subjects and a further four years before all the results were collated and the research published.[10]

They found that men who had survived cancer were about 15 per cent less likely than the average man to have children. Women who had survived cancer were about 5 per cent less likely than the average woman to have children.

The most marked effect on fertility was for men who had received chemotherapy with alkylating agents such as cyclophosphamide, dacarbazine, busulphan, chlorambucil, melphalan or ifosfamide. Treatment with alkylating agents halved the men's chances of having children, although the same drugs did not seem to affect the fertility of women.

Men receiving radiotherapy as boys were also less fertile than the average man. Similarly, women who had received radiotherapy when younger were less fertile than the average woman.

So it is hard to say before treatment starts whether your child is likely to become infertile or not. However your child's doctors should be able to say whether, depending on the drugs used and the doses to be given, it is likely or not.

Are there ways around infertility?

Most treatments for Ewing's sarcoma will not make your son or daughter permanently infertile. But for the forms of treatment that do, it is possible even then to have children, especially if the likelihood of infertility is considered at the time of diagnosis.[11]

Men who are expected to become infertile can donate their sperm to a sperm bank. This is fairly easy—all it requires is for a man to masturbate and collect the sperm in a jar and deliver it, while still warm, to the sperm bank. That sperm is frozen and can be thawed later when required. His partner would then have to undergo artificial insemination with his sperm.

Women who are expected to become infertile can take part in what amounts to an IVF programme. They can have eggs collected which are then fertilised by sperm collected either from the woman's partner or from a sperm bank. The resulting embryos can then be frozen while the woman undergoes treatment for her cancer. Some time later, they can be thawed and implanted into her uterus or fallopian tubes, and she can continue what then becomes a normal pregnancy.

Of course, this sounds fairly easy. There is no guarantee

of success—in fact only a third of women or less who go through this procedure would expect to have a baby. But it is an option that is available, as long as your daughter and her doctors are aware of it.

The ideal situation would be for a woman to be able to freeze eggs. If that could happen, then women who have not settled with their expected partners could still keep eggs but would not have to use a sperm donor. But at the moment, mature eggs can not be frozen successfully.[12]

But it has become possible for women who have become infertile to have children using donated eggs. It is similar to IVF, but instead of using the woman's own eggs, she uses somebody else's. And men who have become infertile can still become a father if their partners have artificial insemination with donor sperm.

But a word of warning about IVF. It involves manipulating the body's hormones, and there is no information on which to judge whether that will have any effect on the cancer. There are no guarantees that delaying treatment until eggs are collected will not make the cancer worse, or that the IVF later on will not make a second cancer more likely. There is no evidence that this will happen, but there are no guarantees that it won't.

Another concern often raised is whether people who have chemotherapy or radiotherapy as children are more likely than average to have children with congenital abnormalities. While this seems to make sense, no studies have shown that it happens. It is likely that being treated for cancer will have no effect on the subsequent chance of having children who are normal.[1]

The whole area of treatment for infertility is complex and changing. But to sum it up, it may help to remember this line: just because you are infertile, it does not mean you can not have children. Technology has made almost anything possible. But many of the technologies are new, and the long-term effects are not yet known.

Other medical problems

Radiation can cause a number of long-term problems. Radiation:
- to the head can cause growth hormone deficiency and short stature;
- to the neck can cause thyroid problems;
- to the mouth, even with minute doses, can cause problems with teeth;
- to or near the spine can cause scoliosis, a curvature of the spine;
- to the face can cause significant facial deformity if doses of more than 30 rads are used;
- can cause cataracts, even some years after radiotherapy, if doses of more than 40 rads are given.[1]

The
Future

A book about what is going on in cancer and its treatment is out of date in some ways as soon as it is published. Much of the information in *Body and Soul* comes from research that was started in the early 1980s, completed in the late 1980s and published in the first year or two of the 1990s. There is a real gap between what the doctors are actually doing, and what we as members of the public can possibly know they are doing.

So by the time you read this book, some of the treatments will have changed, some will have been discarded, and some new ones may have appeared. There is always hope for improvement.

It is probably not wise to look at the future in terms of a 'breakthrough'. People love to use the word 'breakthrough', but it doesn't mean much. Very few advances in medical and scientific research are made by chance—the great majority come down to a hard slog over many years to try to gradually improve what is known and available.

But things do change. Two decades ago, few children survived childhood leukaemia. Now more than 90 per cent survive. Men with testicular cancer have a dramatically improved chance of survival. New ways of giving chemotherapy mean that higher doses can be given which improve the person's chances of being able to tolerate the full course, which then improves their chances of having the chemotherapy work.

There are many different avenues of cancer research that doctors hope and believe will make a difference.

For example, they are working on monoclonal antibodies, which are often described as 'magic bullets'. They are particular parts of cells which can be targeted against other cells. For example, you can make a monoclonal antibody that will go through the bloodstream until it reaches a breast cancer cell and attaches to it.

So if you attach something radioactive, then do an X-ray, you should be able to see exactly where in the body all the breast cancer cells are. This would help to diagnose the extent of the spread of the cancer. And if you attach a form of treatment to the monoclonal antibody, then you should be able to direct the treatment right into the cancer cells. This should mean doctors can use lower doses more effectively.

Specific to Ewing's sarcoma, there is research which can identify very closely the cells which become abnormal. This will help make the diagnosis of Ewing's easier, and will mean treatment can be made more specific.

Gene therapy is also a hot topic in cancer research. Scientists are discovering more and more about the way our genes control the growth of cancer. They are also learning more about how to manipulate these genes, with the hope of being able to switch the faulty ones off. They hope that eventually, if they are dealing with a cancer for which there is a known genetic abnormality, then that cancer gene can be just closed off. The cancer should stop growing.

Doctors and hospitals are continuing to learn that cancer is not just a disease of the body, but that it is part of a life, and part of the lives of many people around the person with the cancer. They are continuing to learn how to improve the support, guidance and information they provide.

They are continuing to learn that it is the person with the cancer who needs to be in control and make the decisions, and have enough information on which to base those decisions, rather than continue with the authoritarian ways of the past.

Of course, some of this progress is still in its early stages. Some of it may come to fruition in the next five or ten years, or some may not happen at all. But we may have brilliant new discoveries which give greater chances to those with cancer, and better care of all involved. The worst that can be said is that things will gradually continue to improve. Beyond that, all you can do is hope.

References

Parents

1 Van Dongen-Melman J. E. W. M. & Sanders-Woudstra J. A. R. Psychosocial aspects of childhood cancer: a review of the literature. *Journal of Child Psychology and Psychiatry* 1986; **27**: 145–80.

2 Carr-Gregg M. & White L. The adolescent with cancer: a psychological overview. *Medical Journal of Australia* 1987; **147**: 496–502.

3 Overholser J. C. & Fritz G. K. The impact of childhood cancer on the family. *Journal of Psychosocial Oncology* 1990; **8**: 71–85.

4 Martinson I. M. & Cohen M. H. Themes from a longitudinal study of family reaction to childhood cancer. *Journal of Psychosocial Oncology* 1988; **6**: 81–98.

5 Beadle G. Personal communication.

6 Cella D. F. Cancer survival: psychosocial and public issues. *Cancer Investigations* 1987; **5**: 59–67.

7 Cornman B. J. Impact of childhood cancer on the family. Unpublished PhD thesis, 1988.

8 Speechley K. N. Surviving childhood cancer: the psychosocial impact on parents. Unpublished PhD thesis. 1987.

Brothers and sisters

1 Carr-Gregg M. & White L. Siblings of pediatric cancer patients: a population at risk. *Medical and Pediatric Oncology* 1987; **15**: 62–8.

2 Chesler M. A., Allswede J. & Barbarin O. O. Voices from the margin of the family: siblings of children with cancer. *Journal of Psychosocial Oncology* 1991; **9**: 19–42.

3 Horwitz W. A. Preschool siblings' adaptation to childhood cancer: competence and development in a family context. Unpublished PhD thesis. 1989.

4 Lauer M. E., Mulhern R. K., Bohne J. B. & Camitta B. M. Children's perceptions of their sibling's death at home or hospital: the precursors of differential adjustment. *Cancer Nursing* 1985; **8**: 21–7.

Coping styles

1 Fritz G. K., Williams J. R. & Amylon M. After treatment ends: psychosocial sequelae in cancer survivors. *American Journal of Orthopsychiatry* 1988; **58**: 552–61.

2 Smith K. E., Ackerson J. P., Blotcky A. D. & Berkow R. Preferred coping styles of pediatric cancer patients during invasive medical procedures. *Journal of Psychosocial Oncology* 1990; **8**: 59–70.

3 Carr-Gregg M. & White L. The adolescent with cancer: a psychological review. *Medical Journal of Australia* 1987; **147**: 496–502.

4 Brock C. Personal communication.

5 Bluebond-Langner M., Perkel D. & Goertzel T. Pediatric cancer patients' peer relationships: the impact of oncology camp experience. *Journal of Psychosocial Oncology* 1991; **9**: 67–80.

6 Varni J. W., Rubenfeld L. A., Talbot D. & Yetoguchi Y.

Stress, social support and depressive symptomatology in children with congenital/acquired limb deficiencies. *Journal of Pediatric Psychology* 1989; **14**: 515–30.

7 Van Dongen-Melman J. E. W. M. & Sanders Woudstra J. A. R. Psychosocial aspects of childhood cancer: a review of the literature. *Journal of Child Psychology and Psychiatry* 1986; **27**: 145–80.

8 Tebbi C. K. & Mallon J. C. Long term psychosocial outcome among cancer amputees in adolescence and early adulthood. *Journal of Psychosocial Oncology* 1987; **5**: 69–82.

9 Welch-McCaffrey D., Hoffman B., Leigh S. A., Loescher L. J. & Meyskens F. L. Surviving adult cancers; 2: psychosocial implications. *Annals of Internal Medicine* 1989; **111**: 517–24.

10 Fritz G. K. & Williams J. R. Issues of adolescent development for survivors of childhood cancer, in S. Chess & M. E. Hertzig (eds) *Annual Progress in Child Psychiatry and Child Development* Brunner/Mazel; New York, 1989.

Teenagers

1 White W. R. The psychosocial impact of cancer in adolescence, in F. W. Gunz & B. W. Stewart (eds) *Cancer Forum* 11, 3. Australian Cancer Society; Sydney, 1987.

2 Carr-Gregg M. & White L. The adolescent with cancer: a psychological overview. *Medical Journal of Australia* 1987; **147**: 496–502.

3 White L. Cancer and adolescence: introduction, overview and the paediatric perspective, in F. W. Gunz & B. W. Stewart (eds) *Cancer Forum.* **11**, 3. Australian Cancer Society, Sydney, 1987.

4 Carr-Gregg M. & Hampson R. A new approach to the psychological care of adolescents with cancer. *Medical Journal of Australia* 1986; **145**: 580–3.

5 Carr-Gregg M. Adolescents with cancer—a consumer report, in F. W. Gunz & B. W. Stewart (eds) *Cancer Forum*, 11, 3, Australian Cancer Society, Sydney, 1987.

6 Carr-Gregg M. R. C. Adolescents with cancer in the

Australian health care system [PhD thesis]. School of Health Administration, University of New South Wales, 1986.

7 McCallum L. & Carr-Gregg M. Adolescents with cancer. *Australian Nurses Journal* 1987; **16**: 39–42.

Long-term effects

1 Mullan F. Seasons of survival: reflections of a physician with cancer. *New England Journal of Medicine* 1985; **313**: 270–3.

2 Hays D. M., Landsverk J., Sallan S. E., Hewett K. D. *et al.* Educational, occupational and insurance status of childhood cancer survivors in their fourth and fifth decades of life. *Journal of Clinical Oncology* 1992; **10**: 1397–406.

3 Nicholson H. S., Mulvihill J. J. & Byrne J. Late effects of therapy in adult survivors of osteosarcoma and Ewing's sarcoma. *Medical and Pediatric Oncology* 1992; **20**: 6–12.

4 Greenberg H. S. & Meadows A. T. Psychosocial impact of cancer survival on school age children and their parents. *Journal of Psychosocial Oncology* 1991; **9**: 43–56.

5 Kazak A. E. & Meadows A. T. Families of young adolescents who have survived cancer: social-emotional adjustment, adaptability and social support. *Journal of Pediatric Psychology* 1989; **14**: 175–91.

6 Carr-Gregg M. The young cancer patient and discrimination. *Australian Nurses Journal* 1989; **18**: 13.

7 Tebbi C. K., Bromberg C. & Piedmonte M. Long term vocational adjustment of cancer patients diagnosed during adolescence. *Cancer* 1989; **63**: 213–18.

8 Welch-McCaffrey D., Hoffman B., Leigh S. A., Loescher L. J. & Meyskens F. L. Surviving adults cancers part 2: psychosocial implications. *Annals of Internal Medicine* 1989; **111**: 517–24.

9 Byrne J., Fears T. R., Steinhorn S. C., Mulvihill J. J. *et al.* Marriage and divorce after childhood and adolescent cancer. *JAMA* 1989; **262**: 2693–9.

10 Byrne J., Mulvihill J. J., Myers M. H. *et al.* Effects of treatment on fertility in long term survivors of childhood or

adolescent cancer. *New England Journal of Medicine* 1987; **317**: 1315–21.

11 Van Dongen-Melman J. E. W. B. & Sanders-Woudstra J. A. R. Psychosocial aspects of childhood cancer: a review of the literature. *Journal of Child Psychology and Psychiatry* 1986; **27**: 145–80.

12 Welch-McCaffrey D. Oncology nurses as cancer patients: an investigative questionnaire. *Oncology Nurses Forum* 1984; **11**: 48.

Sexuality and relationships

1 Dobkin P. L. & Bradley I. Assessment of sexual dysfunction in oncology patients: review, critique and suggestions. *Journal of Psychosocial Oncology* 1991; **9**: 43–74.

2 Fritz G. K. & Williams J. R. Issues of adolescent development for survivors of childhood cancer, in S. Chess & M. E. Hertzig (eds) *Annual Progress in Child Psychiatry and Child Development* Brunner/Mazel, New York, 1989.

3 Schover L. R. *Sexuality and Cancer* 1988, American Cancer Society: New York.

My child is dying

1 Foley G. V. & Whittam E. H. Care of the child dying of cancer: part 1. *Ca—A Cancer Journal for Clinicians* 1990; **40**: 327–54.

2 Kubler-Ross E. *On Death and Dying.* Tavistock, London, 1969.

3 McCallum L. & Carr-Gregg M. Adolescents with cancer. *Australian Nurses Journal* 1987; **16**: 39–42.

4 Carr-Gregg M. & White L. The adolescent with cancer: a psychological overview. *Medical Journal of Australia* 1987; **147**: 496–502.

5 Spinetta J. J., Murphy J. L., Vik P. J., Day J. & Mott M. A. Long-term adjustment in families of children with cancer. *Journal of Psychosocial Oncology* 1988; **6**: 179–91.

Fears and feelings

1 Stern M. & Arenson E. Childhood cancer stereotype: impact on adult perceptions of children. *Journal of Pediatric Psychology* 1989; **14**: 593–605.

2 Stahly G. B. Psychosocial aspects of the stigma of cancer: an overview. *Journal of Psychosocial Oncology* 1988; **6**: 3–27.

3 Welch-McCaffrey D., Hoffman, B., Leigh S. A, Loescher L. J. & Meyskens F. L. Surviving adult cancers; 2: psychosocial implications. *Annals of Internal Medicine* 1989; **111**: 517–24.

4 Smith A. Should a doctor tell the truth when a patient has cancer? *The Times*, May 1976.

5 Foley G. V. & Whittam E. H. Care of the child with cancer, 1: *Ca—A Cancer Journal for Clinicians* 1990; **40**: 327–54.

6. Van Dongen-Melman J. E. W. M. & Sanders-Woudstra J. A. R. Psychosocial aspects of childhood cancer: a review of the literature. *Journal of Child Psychology and Psychiatry* 1986; **27**: 145–80.

7 McKillop W. J., Stewart W. E., Ginsberg A. D. & Stewart S.S. Cancer patients' perceptions of their disease and its treatment. *British Journal of Cancer* 1988; **58**: 355–8.

8 Dunn S. M., Patterson P. U., Butow P. N., Smartt H. H. *et al.* Cancer by another name: a randomised trial in the effects of euphemism and uncertainty in communicating with cancer patients. *Journal of Clinical Oncology* 1993; **11**: 989–96.

9 Friedman G., Florian V. & Zernitsky-Shurka E. The experience of loneliness among young adult cancer patients. *Journal of Psychosocial Oncology* 1989; **7**: 1–15.

Who, What, When and Where

1 Fernbach D. J. & Vietti T. J. (eds). 1989 *Clinical Pediatric Oncology*. 4th edn. Mosby, St Louis.

2 Brown A. P., Fixsen J. A. & Plowman P. N. Local control of Ewing's sarcoma: an analysis of 67 patients. *British Journal of Radiology* 1987; **60**: 261–8.

3 Daugaard S., Sunde L. M., Kamby C., Schiodt T. & Jensen

O. M. Ewing's sarcoma: a retrospective study of prognostic factors and treatment results. *Acta Oncologica* 1987; 26: 281–7.

4 Holly E. A., Aston D. A., Ahn D. K. & Kristiansen J. J. Ewing's bone sarcoma, paternal occupation exposure and other factors. *American Journal of Epidemiology* 1992; **135**: 122–9.

5 Toogood I. R. G. Controversies in the management of primary bone tumours: an Australian perspective. *Medical Journal of Australia* 1988; **188**: 410–12.

6 Singer M. D., Sundaram M. & Naunheim K. Failure of standard imaging techniques in the staging of Ewing's sarcoma. *Journal of Bone and Joint Surgery* 1989. **71–A**, 775–7.

7 Kozlowski K., Campbell J., Beluffi G., Hoeffel J. C. *et al.* Primary bone tumours of the pelvis in childhood, I: Ewing's sarcoma of the ilium, pubis and ischium (report of 30 cases) *Australasian Radiology* 1989; **33**: 354–60.

8 Thomas I. H., Cole W. G., Waters K. D. & Menelaus M. B. Function after partial pelvic resection for Ewing's sarcoma. *Journal of Bone and Joint Surgery* 1987; **69–B**: 271–5.

9 Evans R. E., Nesbit M. E., Gehan E. A., *et al.* Multimodal therapy for the management of localised Ewing's sarcoma of pelvic and sacral bones: a report from the Second Intergroup Study. *Journal of Clinical Oncology* 1991; **9**: 1173–80.

10 Moser R. P., Davis M. J., Gilkey F. W., Kransdorf M. J., *et al.* Primary Ewing sarcoma of the rib. *RadioGraphics* 1990; **10**: 899–914.

11 Kozlowski K., Campbell J., Morris L., Sprague P., *et al.* Primary rib tumours in children: report of 27 cases with short literature review. *Australasian Radiology* 1989; **23**: 210–22.

12 Freeman M. P., Currie C. M., Gray G. F. Jr & Kaye J. J. Ewing sarcoma of the skull with an unusual pattern of reactive sclerosis: MR characteristics. *Journal of Computer Assisted Tomography* 1988; **12**: 143–6.

13 Sneige N. & Batsakis J. G. Ewing's sarcoma of bone and soft tissues. *Annals of Otology, Rhinology and Laryngology* 1989; **98**: 400–2.

14 Arafat A., Ellis G. L. & Adrian J. C. Ewing's sarcoma of the

jaws. *Oral Surgery, Oral Medicine and Oral Pathology* 1983; **55**: 589–96.

15 Siegal G. P., Oliver W. R., Reinus W. R., Gilula L. A. *et al.* Primary Ewing's sarcoma involving the bones of the head and neck. *Cancer* 1987; **60**: 2829–40.

16 Sundaram M., Merenda G. & McGuire M. A skip lesion in association with Ewing sarcoma. *Journal of Bone and Joint Surgery* 1989; **71–A**: 764–8.

17 Kinsella T. J., Lichter A. S., Miser J., Gerber L. & Glatstein E. Local treatment of Ewing's sarcoma: radiation therapy versus surgery. *Cancer Treatment Reports* 1984; **68**: 695–701.

18 Rud N. P., Reiman H. M., Pritchard D. J., Frassica F. J. & Smithson W. A. Extraosseous Ewing's sarcoma: a study of 42 cases. *Cancer* 1989; **64**: 1548–53.

19 O'Keefe F., Lorigan J. G. & Wallace S. Radiological features of extraskeletal Ewing's sarcoma. *British Journal of Radiology* 1990; **63**: 456–60.

20 Sadat A. M. & Ibrahim E. M. Malignant bone tumours in pregnancy: a report of two cases and review of literature. *Indian Journal of Cancer* 1989; **26**: 151–5.

What causes Ewing's sarcoma?

1 Tjalma R. A. Canine bone sarcoma: estimation of relative risk as a function of body size. *Journal of the National Cancer Institute* 1966; **36**: 1137–50.

2 Fraumeni J. F. Stature and malignant tumours of bone in childhood and adolescence. Cancer 1967; **20**: 967–74.

3 National Cancer Institute. *Bone cancer and other sarcomas.* Undated. NCI, Maryland.

4 Broomhall J., May R., Lilleyman J. S. & Milner R. D. G. Height and lymphoblastic leukaemia. *Archives of Diseases in Childhood* 1983; **58**: 300–1.

5 Pendergrass T. W., Foulkes M. A., Robison L. L. & Nesbit M. E. Stature and Ewing's sarcoma in childhood. *American Journal of Pediatric Hematology/Oncology* 1984; **6**: 33–9.

6 Pui C. H., Dodge R. K., George S. L. & Green A. A. Height

at diagnosis of malignancies. *Archives of Diseases in Childhood* 1987; **62**: 495–9.

7 Marsden W. Personal communication.

8 Joyce M. J., Harmon D. C., Mankin H. J., Suit H. D., *et al.* Ewing's sarcoma in female siblings: a clinical report and review of the literature. *Cancer* 1984; **53**: 1959–62.

9 Birch J. M., Hartley A. L., Marsden H. B., Harris M. & Swindell R. Excess risk of breast cancer in mothers of children with soft tissue sarcomas. *British Journal of Cancer* 1984; **49**: 325–31.

10 Hartley A. L., Birch J. M., Marsden H. B. & Harris M. Breast cancer risk in mothers of children with osteosarcoma and chondrosarcoma. *British Journal of Cancer* 1986; **54**: 819–23.

11 Womer R. B. The cellular biology of bone tumours. *Clinical Orthopaedics and Related Research* 1991; **262**: 12–21.

12 Kannourakis G. Personal communication.

13 Davison E. V., Pearson A. D. J., Emslie J., Reid M. M., *et al.* Chromosome 22 abnormalities in Ewing's sarcoma. *Journal of Clinical Pathology* 1989; **42**: 797–9.

14 Holly E. A., Aston D. A., Ahn D. K. & Kristiansen J. J. Ewing's bone sarcoma, paternal occupation exposure and other factors. *American Journal of Epidemiology* 1992; **135**: 122–9.

15 Silcocks P. B. S. & Murrells T. Space-time clustering and bone tumours: application of Knox's method to data from a population-based cancer registry. *British Journal of Cancer* 1987; **40**: 769–71.

16 Glass A. G. & Fraumeni J. F. Epidemiology of bone cancer in children. *Journal of the National Cancer Institute* 1970; **44**: 187–99.

17 Holman C. D. J., Reynolds P. M., Byrne J. J., Trotter J. M. & Armstrong B. K. Possible infectious aetiology in six cases of Ewing's sarcoma in Western Australia. *Cancer* 1983; **52**: 1974–6.

What are our chances?

1 Jurgens H., Exner U., Gadner H., Harms D., *et al.* Multidisciplinary treatment of primary Ewing's sarcoma of bone. *Cancer* 1988; **61**: 23–32.

2 Bacci G., Toni A., Avella M., Manfrini M., *et al.* Long-term results in 144 localised Ewing's sarcoma patients treated with combined therapy. *Cancer* 1989; **63**: 1477–86.

3 Sauer R., Jurgens H., Burgers J. M. V., Dunst J., *et al.* Prognostic factors in the treatment of Ewing's sarcoma: CESS 81. *Radiotherapy and Oncology* 1987; **10**: 101–10.

4 Craft A. W. & Jurgens H. *EICESS 92.* United Kingdom Children's Cancer Study Group, Leicester, 1992.

5 Nesbit M. E., Gehan E. A., Burgert E. O., Vietti T.J., *et al.* Multimodal therapy for the management of primary non-metastatic Ewing's sarcoma of the bone: a long-term follow-up for the first Intergroup study. *Journal of Clinical Oncology* 1990; **8**: 1664–74.

6 Burgert E. O., Nesbit M. E., Garnsey L. A., *et al.* Multimodal therapy for the management of nonpelvic, localised Ewing's sarcoma of bone: Intergroup study IESS-II. *Journal of Clinical Oncology* 1990; **8**: 1514–24.

7 Evans R. G., Nesbit M. E., Gehan E. A., Garnsey L. A., *et al.* Multimodal therapy for the management of localised Ewing's sarcoma of the pelvic and sacral bones: a report from the second Intergroup study. *Journal of Clinical Oncology* 1991; **9**: 1173–80.

8 Kinsella T. J., Miser J. S., Waller B., Venzon D., *et al.* Long term follow-up of Ewing's sarcoma of bone treated with combined modality therapy. *International Journal of Radiation Oncology, Biology and Physics* 1991; **20**: 389–95.

9 Fernbach & Vietti (eds). 1989. *Clinical Pediatric Oncology*, 4th edn. Mosby, St Louis.

10 Meyers P. A. Malignant bone tumours in children: Ewing's sarcoma. *Hematology/Oncology Clinics of North America* 1987; **1**: 667–73.

11 Evans R. G. The four S's of Ewing's sarcoma. *International*

Journal of Radiation Oncology, Biology and Physics 1991; **21**: 1671–3.

12 Gobel V., Jurgens H., Etspuler G., Kemperdick H., *et al.* Prognostic significance of tumor volume in localized Ewing's sarcoma of bone in children and adolescents. *Journal of Cancer Research in Clinical Oncology* 1987; **113**: 187–91.

13 Brown A. P., Fixsen J. A. & Plowman P. N. Local control of Ewing's sarcoma: an analysis of 67 patients. *British Journal of Radiology* 1987; **60**: 261–8.

14 Kannourakis, G. Personal communication.

15 Daugaard S. *et al.* Ewing's sarcoma: a retrospective study of prognostic factors and treatment results. *Acta Oncologica* 1987; **26**: 281–7.

What tests will my child have?

1 Bacci G., Ferrari S., Rosito P., Avella M., *et al.* Sarcoma di Ewing dell'osso: studio anatomoclinico di 424 casi. *Minerva Pediatrica* 1992; **44**: 345–59.

2 Bacci G., Avella M., McDonald D., Toni A., Orlandi M. & Campanacci M. Serum lactate dehydrogenase as a tumor marker in Ewing's sarcoma. *Tumori* 1988; **74**: 649–55.

3 Farley F. A., Healey J. H., Caparros-Sison B., Godbold J., Lane J. M. & Glasser D. B. Lactase dehydrogenase as a tumor marker for recurrent disease in Ewing's sarcoma. *Cancer* 1987; **59**: 1245–8.

4 Erlemann R., Sciuk J., Bosse A., Ritter J., Kusnierz-Glaz C. R., Peters P. E. & Wuisman P. Response of osteosarcoma and Ewing's sarcoma to preoperative chemotherapy: assessment with dynamic and static MR imaging and skeletal scintigraphy. *Radiology* 1990; **175**: 791–6.

5 Frouge C., Vanel D., Coffre C., Couanet D., Contesso G. & Sarrazin D. The role of magnetic resonance imaging in the evaluation of Ewing sarcoma. *Skeletal Radiology* 1988; **17**: 387–92.

6 Silverman J. F. Ancillary studies in FNA of pediatric lesions

(workshop). *XIX International Congress of the International Academy of Pathology*, Madrid. October 1992.

7 Ragg M. *Understanding your thyroid problems.* Gore & Osment: Sydney. 1992.

8 Callen D. F., Smith R. D. & Bourne A. J. Chromosomal analysis in Ewing sarcoma. *Pathology* 1987; **19**: 64–6.

Which treatment and when?

1 Ekert H. *Childhood cancer: understanding and coping* Melbourne 1989.

2 Marsden W. Personal communication.

3 Bacci G., Picci P., Avella M., Ferrari S., *et al.* Neoadjuvant chemotherapy for localised Ewing's sarcoma of bone: experience at the Istituto Ortopedico Rizzoli. *Cancer Journal* 1991; **4**: 335–41.

4 Bacci G., Toni A., Avella M., Manfrini M., *et al.* Multidisciplinary treatment of primary Ewing's sarcoma of bone. *Cancer* 1989; **63**: 1477–86.

Chemotherapy

1 Dresdale A., Bonow R. O. & Wesley R. Prospective evaluation of doxorubicin-induced cardiomyopathy resulting from post-surgical adjuvant treatment of patients with soft tissue sarcomas. *Cancer* 1983; **52**: 51.

2 Kannourakis G. Personal communication.

3 Horowitz M. E., Kinsella T. J., Wexler L. H., Belasco J. *et al.* Total body irradiation and autologous bone marrow transplantation in the treatment of high risk Ewing's sarcoma and rhabdomyosarcoma (in press).

4 Spitzer G. Autotransplantation in solid tumors. *Blood Review* 1991; **5**: 105–11.

5 Yaniv I., Bouffet E., Irle C., Negrier S. *et al.* Autologous bone marrow transplantation in pediatric solid tumors. *Pediatric Hematology and Oncology* 1990; **7**: 35–46.

6 Glasser D. B., Duane K., Lane J. M., Healey J. H. &

Caparros-Sison B. The effects of chemotherapy on growth in the skeletally immature individual. *Clinical Orthopaedics and Related Research* 1991; **262**: 93–100.

7 Kozlowski K., Campbell J., Beluffi G., Hoeffel J. C. *et al.* Primary bone tumours of the pelvis in childhood, I: Ewing's sarcoma of the ilium, pubis and ischium (report of 30 cases) *Australasian Radiology* 1989; **33**: 354–60.

8 Cohen I. J., Loven D., Schoenfeld T., Sandbank J. *et al.* Dactinomycin potentiation of radiation pneumonitis: a forgotten interaction. *Pediatric Hematology and Oncology* 1991; **8**: 187–92.

Radiotherapy

1 Brown et al.

2 Horowitz M. E., Neff J. R. & Kun L. E. Ewing's sarcoma: radiotherapy versus surgery for local control. *Pediatric Clinics of North America* 1991; **38**: 365–80.

3 Goldwein J. W. Effects of radiation therapy on skeletal growth in childhood. *Clinical Orthopedics and Related Research* 1991; **262**: 101–7.

4 Butler M. S., Robertson W. W., Rate W., D'Angio G. J. & Drummond D. S. Skeletal sequelae of radiation therapy for malignant childhood tumors. *Clinical Orthopedics and Related Research* 1990; **251**: 235–40.

Surgery

1 Fernbach D. J. & Vietti, T. J. (eds). 1989 *Clinical Pediatric Oncology* 4th edn. Mosby, St Louis.

2 Van der Eijken J. W. Limb salvage in sarcomas in children. *World Journal of Surgery* 1988; **12**: 318–25.

3 Fernbach D. J. & Vietti, T. J. (eds). 1989 *Clinical Pediatric Oncology* 4th edn. Mosby, St Louis.

4 Marsden W. Personal communication.

5 Lienard D., Rocmans P. & Lejeune F. Resection of lung

metastases from sarcomas. *European Journal of Surgical Oncology* 1989; **15**: 530–34.

6 Lanza L. A. *et al.* The role of resection in the treatment of pulmonary metastases from Ewing's sarcoma. *Journal of Thoracic and Cardiovascular Surgery* 1987; 94–181.

Pain and other problems

1 Bruera E. Symptom control in patients with cancer. *Journal of Psychosocial Oncology* 1990; **8**: 47–73.

2 Portenoy R. K. Pharmacological approaches to the control of cancer pain. *Journal of Psychosocial Oncology* 1990; **8**: 75–107.

3 McGrath P. J., Hsu E., Cappelli M., Luke B. *et al.* Pain from pediatric cancer: a survey of an outpatient oncology clinic. *Journal of Psychosocial Oncology* 1990; **8**: 109–24.

4 Beales J. G. Pain in children with cancer. In J. J. Bonica & V. Ventafridda (eds), *Advances in Pain Research and Therapy* (vol. 2, pp. 89–98). New York, Raven Press, 1979.

Later physical effects of cancer and its treatment

1 Marshall G. Late effects of childhood cancer treatment in adolescents surviving a paediatric malignancy, in F. W. Gunz & B. W. Stewart (eds) *Cancer Forum* **11** (3) Australian Cancer Society, Sydney, 1987.

2 Fernbach D. J. & Vietti T. J. (eds). 1989 *Clinical Pediatric Oncology*. 4th edn. Mosby, St Louis.

3 Butler M. S., Robertson W. W., Rate W., D'Angio G. J. and Drummond D. S. Skeletal sequelae of radiation therapy for malignant childhood tumors. *Clinical Orthopedics and Related Research* 1990; **251**: 235–40.

4 Tucker M. A., D'Angio G. J., Boice J. D., Strong L. C. *et al.* Bone sarcomas linked to radiotherapy and chemotherapy in children. *New England Journal of Medicine* 1987; **317**: 588–93.

5 Daugaard S., Sunde L. M., Kamby C., Schiodt T. and Jensen O. M., Ewing's sarcoma: a retrospective study of prognostic factors and treatment results. *Acta Oncologica* 1987; **26**: 281–7.

6 Boriani S., Picci P., Sudanese A., Toni A. *et al.* Radio-induced sarcomas in survivors of Ewing's sarcoma. *Tumori* 1988; **74**: 543–51.

7 Smith L. M., Cox R. S. & Donaldson S. S. Second cancers in long term survivors of Ewing's sarcoma. *Clinical Orthopedics and Related Research* 1992; **274**: 275–281.

8 Strong L. C., Herson J., Osborne B. M. & Sutow W. W. Risk of radiation-related subsequent malignant tumours in survivors of Ewing's sarcoma. *Journal of the National Cancer Institute* 1979; **62**: 1401.

9 Hubner M. K. Cancer and infertility: longing for life. *Journal of Psychosocial Oncology* 1989; **7**: 1–19.

10 Byrne J., Mulvihill J. J., Myers M. H., Connelly R. R. *et al.* Effects of treatment on fertility in long-term survivors of childhood or adolescent cancer. *New England Journal of Medicine* 1987; **317**: 1315–21.

11 Ford R., Ryan J., Porter R., O'Neill C. *et al.* Preservation of fertility in women undergoing chemotherapy and radio-therapy—the role of embryo cryopreservation and autotransfer. *Cancer Forum* 1989; **13**: 98–100.

12 Saunders D. Personal communication.

Resources

Books

Cancer help: An Australian resource book for patients, helpers, families and friends Henderson and Raymond. Simon & Schuster. 1988.

Something I've never felt before: how teenagers cope with grief Zagdanski. Hill of Content Publishing. 1990.

Too old to cry, too young to die Pendleton (ed). Thomas Nelson Publishers. 1980.

What happened to you happened to me: a book for young people with cancer Kjosness and Rudolph (eds). American Cancer Society. 1983.

When someone in your family has cancer. American Cancer Society. 1984.

Pamphlets

Been there, done that. CanTeen. 1990.

Children with cancer: a handbook for families and helpers

Mager and Parker. American Cancer Society. 1983.
Help yourself: tips for teenagers with cancer. National Cancer
Institute (USA). 1983.

Audio tapes

'Help yourself: tips for teenagers with cancer'. National
Cancer Institute (USA). 1983.

Videos

'Been there, done that'. CanTeen. 1991.
'Teenagers with cancer'. CanTeen. 1985.

Services

There are many many groups, organisations and individuals who are willing to help you. If you need help with emotional support, financial support, travel assistance, accommodation or anything else, some of these groups should be able to help.

CanTeen: The Australian Teenager Cancer Patients Society

Aims: to provide self-help support for teenagers with cancer. CanTeen is based on the idea that one way teenagers with cancer adjust to and cope with their illness is through meeting and supporting other teenagers who are undergoing or who have been through similar experiences.

Services: camps, discussion groups, social outings, 24-hour telephone support, monthly newsletter, penfriend service.

NSW: PO Box 1000
St Pauls 2031
(02) 399 4604 or 399 2106

Hunter (NSW): Social Work Department
Newcastle Mater Hospital
Waratah 2298
(049) 67 9766

Illawarra (NSW): Social Work Department
Wollongong Hospital
Crown St
Wollongong 2500
(042) 20 1295

ACT: GPO Box 316
Curtin 2605
(06) 285 3070

Vic: c/- Australian Red Cross Society (Vic)
171 City Rd
South Melbourne 3205
(03) 616 9972

SA: GPO Box 1093
Adelaide 5001
(08) 267 7488

Tas: PO Box 475
Launceston 7250
(003) 31 6433

WA: Denis St
Subiaco 6008
(09) 388 3594

NT: PO Box 42719
Casuarina 0811
(089) 27 4888

Qld: PO Box 168
    Stone's Corner 4120
    (07) 397 0604

Camp Quality

Aims: to provide camping experience and support
programmes for children with cancer and their families.
Volunteers have professional guidance when needed.

Service: run 2–3 camps each year.

NSW: 14 Taylor St
    West Pennant Hills 2120
    (02) 872 5454

Hunter (NSW): 171 Northcott Dr
            Adamstown Heights 2289
            (049) 57 5443

Illawarra (NSW): 54 Gwinganna Ave
            Kiama 2533
            (042) 21 1967

ACT: 113 Darwinia Terrace
    Rivett 2611
    (06) 288 4554

Vic: PO Box 409
    Heidelberg 3084
    (03) 459 4437

SA: 11 Cummins St
    Novar Gardens 5040
    (08) 295 1220

Tas: GPO Box 1758T
    Hobart 7001
    (002) 44 7456

WA: 15 Currawong Dr
     Gooseberry Hill 6076
     (09) 293 2140

Qld: GPO Box 1017
     Springwood 4127
     (07) 208 7482

Nth Qld: PO Box 1538
     Townsville 4810
     (077) 74 0181

CanYA

For people aged 20–35 who are undergoing treatment for or who have had cancer. Regular meetings, newsletters and hospital and home visits provide opportunities for young adults with cancer to share experiences and feelings.

PO Box 511
St Leonards 2065
(02) 438 7176 (ask for Christina Brock)
(02) 357 1112 (leave message)

Childhood Cancer Association
PO Box 138
Henley Beach SA 5022
(08) 388 9434

National Association for Loss and Grief

Aims: To encourage and promote professional and community education in areas of loss and grief. To encourage investigation, study and research of the human experience of loss and grief. To promote and organise cooperation and coordination in the achievement of the above.

PO Box 79
Turramurra 2074
(02) 499 5279

Australian Capital Territory Cancer Society
PO Box 509
Canberra 2601
(06) 243 2111

The Queensland Cancer Fund
PO Box 201
Spring Hill 4000
(07) 257 1155

Northern Territory Anti-Cancer Foundation
GPO Box 718
Darwin 5794
(089) 81 3556

Anti-Cancer Foundation of the Universities of South Australia
PO Box 160
North Adelaide 5006
(08) 228 5070

Cancer Foundation of Western Australia
42 Ord St
West Perth 6005
(09) 321 6224

Tasmanian Cancer Committee
c/- GPO Box 191B
Hobart 7001
(002) 30 6315

Tasmanian Cancer Support and Information Service
Liverpool St
Hobart 7000

Anti-Cancer Council of Victoria
1 Rathdowne St
Carlton South 3035
(03) 662 3300

New South Wales Cancer Council
151 Dowling St
Woolloomooloo 2011
(02) 334 1900

Australian Cancer Society
GPO Box 4708
Sydney 2001
(02) 267 1944

Clinical Oncology Society of Australia
GPO Box 4708
Sydney 2001
(02) 267 1944

Cancer Help Line (SA)
(08) 267 5222 or (008) 188 070

Hospice/palliative care contact

ACT: Chief social worker
       Woden Valley Hospital
       Garran 2606
       (06) 281 0433

Qld: Dr John Cavenagh
       Hospice Unit
       Mount Olivet Hospital
       411 Main St
       Kangaroo Point 4169
       (07) 391 8811

SA: c/- the Anti-Cancer Foundation of the
       Universities of SA
       PO Box 55
       Rundle Mall PO
       Adelaide 5001
       (08) 227 5070

WA: Dr Rosalie Shaw
       Palliative care unit
       Repatriation General Hospital
       Hollywood 6009
       (09) 386 0011

Tas: Hospice Care Association of Southern Tasmania
       The Coach House
       St John's Hospital
       30 Cascade Rd
       South Hobart 7004
       (002) 23 5042

Vic: Victorian Association of Hospice Care Programs
       c/- Melbourne City Mission Hospice Program
       10 Church St
       Fitzroy North 3068
       (03) 489 9666

The Compassionate Friends

Aims: To provide comfort and support to parents of
children who have died at any age from any cause. To
enrol parents or family members of children who have

died so that they can support other children dying from any cause.

Services: Bi-monthly newsletter, telephone counselling, drop-in centres in some states, regional contacts in some states.

NSW: Room 307
381 Pitt St
Sydney 2000
(02) 267 6962

WA: (09) 227 5698

Vic: (03) 882 3355

Qld: (075) 52 3142

SA: (08) 294 6700

ACT: (06) 254 6226
(06) 286 6134
(06) 248 5471

Tas: (002) 55 2145

NT: (089) 27 8416

Transport

Assistance with transport is quite limited. Check with:
• your local hospital (social work department)
• volunteer groups such as Rotary or Lions Club
• local church groups
• local community health centre

Social security benefits

A carer's pension is available to a relative who personally provides their 'severely handicapped' relative with constant care and attention at home. To be 'severely handicapped', the person must need help to do things like prepare food, eat, dress, wash, move about the home.

To claim a carer's pension, you will probably need a medical report from your relative's doctor. A carer's pension is subject to an income and assets test.

Other people/organisations who may be able to help

If you have no luck with one of the organisations listed above, and the list is by no means exhaustive, then there are many other people who can either provide help or tell you how to get it. These include:
• hospitals
• hospices
• general practitioners
• specialists
• home nursing services
• social workers
• occupational therapists
• ministers of religion
• interpreter services
• cancer support groups
• community health centres
• Meals on Wheels

Index